Precepting Medical Students in the Office

Precepting Medical Students in the Office ▪ ▪ ▪

▪ ▪ ▪ Edited by

Paul M. Paulman, M.D.
Jeffrey L. Susman, M.D.
Cheryl A. Abboud, M.P.A.

The Johns Hopkins University Press
Baltimore and London

© 2000 The Johns Hopkins University Press
All rights reserved. Published 2000
Printed in the United States of America on acid-free paper
9 8 7 6 5 4 3 2 1

The Johns Hopkins University Press
2715 North Charles Street
Baltimore, Maryland 21218-4363
www.press.jhu.edu

Library of Congress Cataloging-in-Publication Data will be found
at the end of this book.
A catalog record for this book is available from the British Library.

ISBN 0-8018-6366-X (pbk.)

To all our children:
Roger, Katie, Katie, Dan, Ben, and Sarah.

And a special thanks to Suellen Miller
for all her help in making this work possible.

Contents

III. Clinical Teaching

VI. Legal and Ethical Aspects of Precepting

VII. Faculty Benefits and Resources

Foreword

The young man sat attentively at the knee of Maimonides, the famous Hebrew physician. Even though his practice included the Egyptian royal court and an entire suburb of Cairo, Maimonides still felt it important to be a teacher because this was a tradition that went far back into history.

Since the fifth century B.C., the training of new physicians has been accomplished through an apprenticeship in which the neophyte receives instruction, does menial tasks, and participates in the care of patients at the bedside. This concept was so important to early physicians that it was incorporated into the Oath of Hippocrates.

I swear by Apollo, the physician, by Aesculapius, by Hygeia, by Panacea, and by all the Gods and Goddesses, calling them to witness that according to my ability and judgment, I will in every particular keep this, my oath and covenant, to regard him who teaches this art equally with my parents, to share my substance, and if he be in need, to relieve his necessities, to regard his offspring equally with my brethren, and to teach his art if they shall wish to learn it, without fee or stipulations, to impart a knowledge by precept, by lecture, and by every other mode of instruction to my sons, to the sons of my teacher, and to pupils who are bound by stipulation and oath, according to the law of medicine but to no other.

From Hippocrates, *"Oath," translated by W. H. S. Jones in the Loeb Classical Library, Cambridge: Harvard University Press, 1923*

Medical knowledge and training have evolved dramatically over the centuries, but the tradition of dedicated physicians sharing their knowledge, skills, experience, and wisdom with the next generation of young medical students is still vital. Much of today's medical training is of a technical nature, but in reality physicians are as much artists as technicians, and the art of medicine is a skill that cannot be learned in a classroom. As Hippocrates put it a long time ago, the doctor who despises the knowledge acquired by the ancients is foolish.

Today many medical schools have established departments of family medicine, and this has greatly increased the demand for teachers. Medical schools have turned to community preceptors to provide their students with "real world" training experiences in family medicine.

In the past decade, there has been a great increase in the demands on family physicians. With the advent of managed care and other economic considerations, physicians are under increased stress. This stress is nothing new, as evidenced by a statement from Hippocrates's time, 2,500 years ago: "Life is short and art long; the crisis fleeting, experience perilous, and decision difficult. The physician must be prepared not only to do what is right himself, but also to make the patient, the attendants, and externals cooperate."

A recurring theme heard wherever physicians gather is "practice just isn't any fun anymore." There are many competing demands for our time and attention, from patients, payers, and, of course, the government. Doctors feel as if they're working harder for less: less pay, less fun, less control, less collegiality.

Despite all these changes, medicine continues to be a very special profession with wonderful ties that bind us together as practitioners of our art. Acting as preceptors, we can share our knowledge and experience; and the preceptorship can be a powerful stimulus to our own lifelong learning. David Riesman wrote that if you want to get the fullest enjoyment out of medicine you should be a student all your life. It is always refreshing to interact with excited and enthusiastic young people because they have not been jaded by cynicism and the stresses of running a modern medical practice. In *The Fall*, Albert Camus says that we are forgiven for our happiness and successes only if we generously consent to share them.

In his *Nicomachean Ethics*, Aristotle said that happiness depends on ourselves. Precepting can be a means of putting joy back into our medical lives. Like most of the special things in life, it takes time, patience, and effort, but the rewards are great. Besides, it is our sacred duty.

Stuart P. Embury, M.D.
Practicing Physician, Holdrege, Nebraska

Preface

Community physician preceptors are the unsung heroes of medical education. As medical care focuses increasingly on the ambulatory arena and teaching outside the academic medical center, community preceptors have become the backbone of many medical schools. Community preceptorships provide tremendous opportunities for students: increased independence and autonomy, more hands-on experience, and powerful mentoring relationships. Indeed, many medical students rate their community rotations as their best experience in medical school.

While the clinical wisdom of community preceptors is unsurpassed, many have had no formal training in educating their students. The goal of this book is to fill this gap. We hope this manual will offer practical insights into how to accomplish everything from orienting a student to providing effective feedback. Chapters have been kept brief and focused. Each chapter is meant to stand alone and act as a ready reference on a particular topic; thus, you will find redundancy if you read this entire book in one sitting. No matter what your approach, our hope is that you will find these "pearls" from experienced educators to be accessible and practical.

There are many parallels between caring for patients and teaching health care professionals. You take a history (a student's educational background and needs), perform an examination (observe a student's performance), arrive at a diagnosis (assess that student's performance), and develop a therapeutic plan (provide feedback and suggestions for continuing improvement). Like your patients, students benefit greatly from your efforts and value your commitment for years to come. We salute you, the community teachers who make our preceptorships so successful.

Contributors

Cheryl A. Abboud, M.P.A., Administrator, Department of Pathology and Microbiology, University of Nebraska Medical Center, Omaha, Nebraska

Laurence C. Bauer, M.S.W., M.Ed., Assistant Professor, Department of Family Medicine, Wright State University, Dayton, Ohio

Dan Benzie, M.D., Clinical Associate Professor, Department of Family Medicine, University of Minnesota, Duluth, Minnesota

William Bondurant, M.D., Associate Clinical Professor, Department of Family Medicine, University of Oklahoma, Oklahoma City, Oklahoma

James L. Brand, M.D., Associate Professor and Medical Director, Family Medicine Center, Department of Family and Preventive Medicine, University of Oklahoma Health Sciences Center, Oklahoma City, Oklahoma

JoAnn M. Carpenter, M.D., Associate Clinical Professor, Family Medicine Center, Department of Family and Preventive Medicine, University of Oklahoma Health Sciences Center, Oklahoma City; Practicing Physician, Ada, Oklahoma

Alexander W. Chessman, M.D., Associate Professor, Department of Family Medicine, Medical University of South Carolina, Charleston, South Carolina

Lili Church, M.D., Assistant Professor, Department of Family Medicine, University of Washington, Seattle, Washington

Joyce Copeland, M.D., Clinical Assistant Professor, Duke University Medical Center, Durham, North Carolina

Gregory A. Doyle, M.D., Associate Professor, Department of Family Medicine, West Virginia University Health Sciences Center, Morgantown, West Virginia

Susan Epstein, M.P.A., Chief, Division of Community Health, Department of Community and Family Medicine, Duke University Medical Center, Durham, North Carolina

Julea Garner, M.D., Family Physician, Private Practice, Glencoe, Arkansas

Thomas Greer, M.D., M.P.H., Associate Professor, Department of Family Medicine, University of Washington, Seattle, Washington

Joseph Hobbs, M.D., Professor and Chair, Department of Family Medicine, Medical College of Georgia, Augusta, Georgia

Cynthia A. Irvine, M.Ed., Department of Family and Community Medicine, University of California, San Francisco, California

A. Patrick Jonas, M.D., Clinical Associate Professor, Department of Family Medicine, Wright State University, Dayton, Ohio

Norman B. Kahn Jr., M.D., Vice President, Education and Science, American Academy of Family Physicians, Kansas City, Missouri

Katherine C. Krause, M.D., Clinical Professor and Vice Chair, Department of Family Practice and Community Medicine, University of Pennsylvania Medical School, Philadelphia, Pennsylvania

Paula S. Krauser, M.D., M.A., Clinical Associate Professor, Department of Family Medicine, University of Medicine and Dentistry of New Jersey–Robert Wood Johnson Medical School, New Brunswick, New Jersey

Harold Krueger, Administrator, Chadron Community Hospital, Chadron, Nebraska

Walter L. Larimore, M.D., Clinical Associate Professor of Family Medicine, University of South Florida, Tampa, Florida; Private Practice, Heritage Family Physicians, Kissimee, Florida

Steven L. Lawrence, M.D., Associate Professor, Department of Family and Community Medicine, Medical College of Wisconsin, Milwaukee, Wisconsin

Michael K. Magill, M.D., Professor and Chair, Department of Family and Preventive Medicine, University of Utah School of Medicine, Salt Lake City, Utah

Mary Ann Manners, M.S.P.H., Instructor, Department of Family Medicine, University of Nebraska Medical Center, Omaha, Nebraska

Christine C. Matson, M.D., Associate Dean for Education, Eastern Virginia Medical School, Norfolk, Virginia

Anne McCarthy, M.D., Resident, Moses H. Cone Memorial Hospital, Greensboro, North Carolina

Lee Montgomery, M.D., Family Physician, Private Practice, Fulton, Mississippi

William K. Mygdal, Ed.D., Director, Faculty Development Center of Texas, Waco, Texas

Laeth Nasir, M.D., Associate Professor, Department of Family Medicine, University of Nebraska Medical Center, Omaha, Nebraska

James MacColl Nicholson, M.D., Clinical Assistant, University of Pennsylvania, Philadelphia, Pennsylvania

David Olson, M.D., Associate Clinical Professor of Family Medicine, Family Health Plan, Elm Grove, Wisconsin

Audrey A. Paulman, M.D., Assistant Clinical Professor, Department of Family Medicine, University of Nebraska Medical Center, Omaha, Nebraska

Paul M. Paulman, M.D., Professor and Predoctoral Director, Department of Family Medicine, University of Nebraska Medical Center, Omaha, Nebraska

Jessica Pierce, Ph.D., Assistant Professor, Department of Preventive and Societal Medicine, University of Nebraska Medical Center, Omaha, Nebraska

Gayle Primrose, Administrator, Boone County Health Center, Albion, Nebraska

Rick E. Ricer, M.D., Professor and Director of Predoctoral Education, Department of Family Medicine, University of Cincinnati College of Medicine, Cincinnati, Ohio

Richard G. Roberts, M.D., J.D., Professor, Department of Family Medicine, University of Wisconsin Medical School, Madison, Wisconsin

Joseph E. Scherger, M.D., M.P.H., Professor and Chair, Department of Family Medicine, and Associate Dean of Primary Care, University of California College of Medicine, Irvine, California

Peter Schludermann, M.D., Associate Clinical Professor, Department of Family Medicine, Oregon Health Sciences University, Portland, Oregon

L. Peter Schwiebert, M.D., Professor and Director of Predoctoral Education, Department of Family and Preventive Medicine, University of Oklahoma Health Sciences Center, Oklahoma City, Oklahoma

Kent J. Sheets, Ph.D., Associate Professor and Director of Educational Development, Department of Family Medicine, University of Michigan Medical School, Ann Arbor, Michigan

Roger C. Shenkel, M.D., Family Physician, Grand Junction, Colorado

William B. Shore, M.D., Professor, Department of Family and Community Medicine, University of California, San Francisco, California

Mark Simon, M.D., Resident, Exempla St. Joseph Hospital, Denver, Colorado

Jeffrey A. Stearns, M.D., Associate Professor, Department of Family and Community Medicine, University of Illinois College of Medicine, Rockford, Illinois

David J. Steele, Ph.D., Associate Professor and Director, Integrated Clinical Experience Program, Department of Family Medicine, University of Nebraska Medical Center, Omaha, Nebraska

Keith Stelter, M.D., Assistant Professor, Department of Family Medicine, University of Minnesota, Minneapolis, Minnesota

Curtis C. Stine, M.D., Associate Professor, Department of Family Medicine, University of Colorado School of Medicine, Denver, Colorado

Marian R. Stuart, Ph.D., Clinical Professor, Department of Family Medicine, University of Medicine and Dentistry of New Jersey–Robert Wood Johnson Medical School, New Brunswick, New Jersey

Jeffrey L. Susman, M.D., Director, Department of Family Medicine, University of Cincinnati

Anita D. Taylor, M.A.Ed., Associate Professor, Department of Family Medicine, Oregon Health Sciences University, Portland, Oregon

William L. Toffler, M.D., Professor, Department of Family Medicine, Oregon Health Sciences University, Portland, Oregon

Richard P. Usatine, M.D., Associate Clinical Professor, Department of Family Medicine, University of California, Los Angeles, California

Daniel J. Van Durme, M.D., Associate Professor, Department of Family Medicine, University of South Florida, Tampa, Florida

Patrick T. Waters, D.O., Clinical Assistant Professor, Department of Family and Community Medicine, University of Pennsylvania School of Medicine, Philadelphia, Pennsylvania; Practicing Community Physician

Neal Whitman, Ed.D., Professor, Department of Family and Preventive Medicine, University of Utah School of Medicine, Salt Lake City, Utah

■ I

Introduction to Community-Based Precepting

■ 1

The History and Value of Preceptorships

William K. Mygdal, Ed.D.

Historically, the route to becoming a physician was all about mentoring, learning, and seeing—a didactic exposure to the protocols of medicine and the relationships on which success-ful medical practice depended. Physician-teachers set standards and expectations and served as mentors day in and day out. . . . Today we're still modeling. As teachers, part of our job is to be the role models and mentors that will shape the character of tomorrow's medical profession.

Nancy Wilson Dickey, M.D.
Family Physician and President of the
American Medical Association

Key Points

- Preceptorships help connect medical students and teachers, creating powerful role models.
- Preceptorships provide useful knowledge and skills, particularly in areas in which most health science centers are deficient.
- Preceptorships challenge students to think in new ways and integrate their training.

Historical Perspective

The major changes in undergraduate medical education during the past decade, which include a renewed empha-sis on preceptorships, the introduction of problem-based learning, and greater reliance on ambulatory training, can be seen in part as attempts to reconnect students with their teachers and to provide the human contact and interaction that is so important to effective learning. American medicine has in fact a long preceptorial tradition, beginning with three-year apprenticeships during the colonial era. During the nineteenth century, medical schools relied on private practitioners for most of their instruction. Reform of medical education and the infusion of massive research funding following World War II led to the present era's very much larger full-time medical school faculties and a resulting deemphasis of preceptorships (Starr, 1982). Current efforts to reinvigorate the preceptorship tradition, led by family physicians, seek to reestablish the connection between preceptor and student and to encourage physicians to become the role models and mentors who will, as Nancy Dickey notes, "shape the character of tomorrow's medical profession" (Dickey, 1997).

The Value of Community-Based Preceptorships

Preceptorships Help Connect Medical Students and Medical Teachers

Medical schools today are large and complex. Their curricula consist of numerous courses and rotations taught by a large and changing cadre of basic scientists and clinicians. At the preclinical level, students typically learn in large groups, attending lectures and participating in laboratory experiences. While completing their clinical rotations, they are introduced to various medical disciplines every month or two and must repeatedly learn to work in new environments with different teachers. A frequent result of this complex curriculum is that students' learning experiences become fragmented. Apart from their community-based preceptorships, students have little opportunity for extended day-to-day personal contact with practicing clinicians and little occasion to establish the mentor relationships so eloquently cited by Dr. Dickey.

Preceptorships Provide Students with Effective Role Models

During the course of a community preceptorship (typically lasting one month to six weeks), the student and practicing physician will get to know each other well and observe each other more closely than in any other relationship in the student's medical school experience. This extended contact enables the student to observe how the preceptor's practice operates, permits observations of the preceptor's relationship with patients, and enables the student to see how the preceptor solves clinical problems. Indeed, a study by Epstein et al. (1998) found that "active observation" was the most common mode of learning during preceptorships. I recently asked two students what observations had most impressed them during these experiences. One commented that "I saw that my preceptor's patients didn't just like her, they *loved* her," and another said he valued most observing his preceptor's daily routine and his "contagious enthusiasm" for the practice of medicine (C. Mygdal and P. Mygdal, pers. comm., Oct. 24, 1998).

Finally, successful preceptorships involve active learning by the student and the assumption of increasing levels of responsibility for patient care (Biddle, Riesenberg, and Darcy, 1996). By providing opportunities for ample "hands-on" practice, preceptors help students move from the domain of abstract and theoretical knowledge to the application of that knowledge to patient care.

Preceptorships Help Reestablish Balance between Hospital and Ambulatory Experiences

Students receive invaluable grounding in clinical medicine during their rotations in the academic medical center. However, through preceptorships they learn to work with healthy ambulatory patients whose medical problems and health concerns represent those of the population as a whole. Preceptorships also give students exposure to primary care specialists, thereby enabling them to choose a specialty on the basis of their own experience. Given the broad consensus among the public, health policy planners, and legislators that the United States needs more generalist physicians, preceptorships are an essential educational strategy for developing greater student interest in the primary care disciplines.

Preceptorships Provide Both Challenge and Support

Medical students face a daunting learning task: They must assimilate and apply huge amounts of new information in frequently changing settings and must often rethink, modify, and reconfigure what they have previously learned. They rapidly acquire new procedural and inter-actional skills and emulate the professional attitudes and values of their teachers. It is not surprising that many students find medical training demanding and stressful. In this context, the preceptor can provide much-needed confirmation, encouragement, and support. One of the students with whom I talked told me that "a compliment from my preceptor could keep me going for a week!" (P. Mygdal, pers. comm., Oct. 24, 1998).

The preceptor can make an enormous contribution by getting to know the student, confirming the student's knowledge and skill, correcting mistakes or misunderstandings, and providing challenge and support as students start to assume their new professional identities as physicians. Preceptorships allow students to see "the light at the end of the tunnel." They come to realize that eventually their own training will end and they will establish a satisfying practice. In many cases, the mutual respect between preceptor and student leads to a redirection of the student's choice of specialty or mentoring relationship.

The Rewards of Precepting

Physicians who become preceptors soon realize that they are working with extremely bright learners. They often cite the stimulation of interacting with their students as one of their principal satisfactions. Students bring new knowledge to the preceptor's practice. They ask "why," challenge assumptions, and lend prestige to the preceptor and the preceptor's practice in the eyes of patients. Many physicians cite precepting activities as a beneficial stimulus in helping them keep abreast of new medical information and revisiting knowledge and skills that have atrophied. Preceptorships enable students to satisfy their hunger to experience "real medicine," to interact with and touch patients, to apply their learning, and to connect with a valued teacher and mentor. When they work right, preceptorships are a highly satisfying experience for both teacher and learner.

References

Biddle, W. B., Riesenberg, L. A., and Darcy, P. A. 1996. Medical students' perceptions of desirable characteristics of primary care teaching sites. *Family Medicine* 28:629–33.

Dickey, N. W. 1997. Blanchard memorial lecture. Society of Teachers of Family Medicine Annual Spring Conference. Boston, Mass.

Epstein, R. M., Cole, D. R., Gawinski, B. A., Piotrowski-Lee, S., and Ruddy, N. B. 1998. How students learn from community-based preceptors. *Archives of Family Medicine* 7:149–54.

Starr, P. 1982. *The Social Transformation of American Medicine.* New York: Basic Books.

▪ 2

How Do I Get Involved in Precepting?

Paul M. Paulman, M.D.

Key Points

- Becoming a preceptor is as easy as contacting your local health professional school or residency program.
- The American Academy of Family Physicians (AAFP), Association of American Medical Colleges (AAMC), Society of Teachers of Family Medicine (STFM), and other professional societies are ready sources of information about precepting.
- Your local area health education center (AHEC) may also have excellent resources.

The trend in undergraduate medical education in the past decade has been to increase medical students' exposure to community practice via community rotations. There are more than 120 medical and osteopathic colleges in the United States that require community clinical rotations in one or more disciplines. More than 50 medical and osteopathic colleges are planning or offering required community rotations for preclinical students in the first two years of school. Many of these community rotations require a one-to-one community faculty-to-student ratio. These factors have resulted in a marked increase in the need for community preceptors in many disciplines in virtually all areas of the United States. Community preceptors are particularly needed in inner-city urban and rural areas as well as in "special circumstance" practices such as Indian Health Service sites and prisons. While community preceptors are needed in all medical disciplines, the greatest need exists in the generalist disciplines of family medicine, general internal medicine, and general pediatrics.

If you want to become a community preceptor, your best information sources are:

1. Your area medical or osteopathic college. You should speak to your department chair or department's director of predoctoral education. The Association of American Medical Colleges keeps a current list of medical colleges in the United States. The American Association of Colleges of Osteopathic Medicine (AACOM) maintains a list of osteopathic colleges in the United States.

   Association of American Medical Colleges
   2450 N Street, NW
   Washington, D.C. 20037-1126
   (202) 828-0400

   American Association of Colleges
      of Osteopathic Medicine
   5550 Friendship Boulevard, Suite 300
   Chevy Chase, Md. 20815-7201
   (301) 968-4100

2. Your specialty society, via national, state, or local chapters. Some specialty societies have a particular interest in assisting community preceptors.

   American Academy of Family Physicians
   11400 Tomahawk Creek Parkway, Suite 540
   Leawood, Kans. 66211
   (800) 274-2237

Society of Teachers of Family Medicine
11400 Tomahawk Creek Parkway, Suite 540
Leawood, Kans. 66211
(800) 274-2237

American College of Physicians /
    American Society of Internal Medicine
190 North Independence Mall West
Philadelphia, Pa. 19106-1572
(800) 523-1546

American Academy of Pediatrics (AAP)
141 Northwest Point Boulevard
Elk Grove Village, Ill. 60007-1098
(800) 433-9016

3. Your area health education center. These federally
funded agencies may offer or coordinate community
rotations for medical students.

Area Health Education Center
Department of Health and Human Services
Division of Medicine, Room 9A27
Parklawn Building
5600 Fishers Lane
Rockville, Md. 20857
(301) 443-6950

4. The American Medical Student Association (AMSA).
This group maintains a list of student community
rotations, and may be a resource for finding students
in your area who are interested in community
rotations.

American Medical Student Association
1902 Association Drive
Reston, Va. 20191-9831
(800) 767-2266

Many community physicians have started precepting by inviting one or more medical students from the physician's community or practice. This is probably the best way to ensure a pleasant first experience with students in your office.

Before you start teaching medical students in your practice, be aware that costs (both time and money) are involved. Your patients and staff will need to make certain adjustments, and visiting students require logistic support and supervision. Despite these potential drawbacks, thousands of community physicians find that the intellectual stimulation and satisfaction of precepting far outweigh any problems encountered in teaching medical students. With careful planning and preparation, you'll find that teaching students in your practice will be rewarding and enjoyable.

▪ 3

Pitfalls of Precepting

William L. Toffler, M.D., Anita D. Taylor, M.A.Ed., and Peter Schludermann, M.D.

Key Points
- Precepting medical students is an enjoyable activity.
- There are pitfalls of precepting that can be anticipated and often avoided or altered to improve the teaching process.

Teaching medical students in your office can be rewarding. However, there are conditions that may interfere with the teaching process. Here are several points to consider.

Don't precept a student when you are overcommitted and stressed. The last thing students need to see are role models who reflect exhaustion, irritability, or even depression. Stressed preceptors may be tempted to vent with students. The students do not know how to put the stress of the preceptor in perspective and this puts an unfair burden on them (a student shouldn't be used as a therapist).

Don't hesitate to discuss mutual expectations for the preceptorship. It is unfair to be upset with students' performance when you have not discussed rotation goals and objectives. Also, students inevitably come with hopes and expectations about the preceptorship. You might simply ask, "By the end of six weeks, what measurable skills or knowledge do you wish to acquire or improve that you don't possess now?"

Don't try to teach too much. One of the hardest things to do is to avoid lecturing. All learners have limited attention spans and are unlikely to retain more than a fraction of what is said. Conveying one or two important pieces of information per patient will result in dozens of new insights for the student each day. If time is limited and your student has questions about a substantial issue, you can suggest discussing it over lunch or at the end of the day.

Don't have students see everything you do. It is important to give students specific tasks while you see other patients, dictate, use the telephone, or visit with a patient privately. Such variety tends to stimulate and energize. Having the students simply follow you about encourages passivity. Possible tasks for the student may include observing the lab technician for a couple of hours or reading up on a problem seen in the clinic.

Don't make assumptions about your students' knowledge. Students come from a variety of backgrounds and often have significant expertise in some areas. In addition, changes in curricula may provide earlier clinical experience than was the case in the past. Your students may expect a higher degree of participation than was true when you trained in medical school. Don't assume that all students have the same level of knowledge and experience, especially early in the clinical years.

Don't fail to review your student's work. Time may not allow a full discussion of things a student may want to share. The student will learn, when asked, to summarize the important points of an interaction with a patient.

Don't assume that documentation by students is adequate or appropriate. Even if the basic content is correct, the tone and focus of the student's visit note may vary significantly from your preferred documentation. In addition, some third-party payers, such as Medicare, have rules about documentation by medical students. When in doubt, check with specific carriers in your region. If uncertain, dictate your own note. Review student documentation for personal judgment or bias and medical-legal risk issues.

Avoid giving the impression that you'd "rather not have" the student. Students are generally very sensitive to your needs and will likely be receptive or even appreciative that you communicate your concerns directly. If you feel pressed for time on a given day and find it difficult to cope with a learner underfoot, you might introduce the student to an associate, partner, or one of the staff who might be able to work with the student for a specified interval. Alternatively, simply ask the student to come back on a different day when it is less likely that conditions will be as stressful. Share with the student your need to keep the clinic schedule moving or to step in with difficult or time-consuming patients.

Avoid misrepresentation. In general, students don't mind being introduced as learners, but sometimes can feel awkward, embarrassed, or guilty when they are introduced as "doctor." In addition, patients may feel misled (or even resentful) if they subsequently learn the true status of the medical student.

Don't fail to assess student competence. Ideally, discussion of a student's performance should take place apart from the exam room and out of the presence of the patient. Otherwise, either the patient or the student may well feel "put on the spot."

Avoid subtle "putdowns" of the student in front of the patient. Although appropriate questioning and use of a Socratic method may be effective in some circumstances, these may not always represent the best approach. Strive to acknowledge significant strengths and experience that the student demonstrates.

Don't fail to review your student's homework. Students can come to resent a constant stream of suggestions for self-study, however well intended, when there is no follow-up or closure of multiple earlier directives.

Don't fail to keep your commitments. If a student expects to work with you and you are unavoidably delayed, make an effort to communicate this information to the student. Think of your own consternation when you are asked to wait for even a few minutes without any clear explanation. Also, make yourself available so the student can inform you of his or her delays and schedule changes.

Don't hesitate to mention issues that are a source of significant annoyance. A student's behavior, dress, or even personal hygiene may cause you some irritation or frustration. We all try to learn sensitivity and tolerance of diversity, especially with religious or cultural differences. Some issues may interfere with the quality of precepting or patient care. If there are specific concerns, never ignore them by conveying to the student that he or she is doing fine. The last thing a student wants is to be reassured that all is well, only to learn of specific behavioral deficiencies long after the rotation is completed. One way of approaching behavioral issues might be to express your feeling directly, but with sensitivity. For example, if you have concerns about dress, you could say, "I need to share my discomfort with you about your appearance in the office. While it would be fine for you to wear those sandals during your free time, they are not professional-looking enough for my office and I would appreciate it if you wore closed shoes."

Having a student in your practice requires extra planning and attention to details. With such effort, preceptors can avoid these pitfalls.

Characteristics and Needs
of Learners

■ 4

What Medical Students Want and Need from a Preceptorship

Lee Montgomery, M.D.

Key Points
- Preceptors should explicitly assess student needs and wants.
- Timely, specific, and balanced feedback enhances the learning experience.

Community preceptors provide an exciting opportunity for enthusiastic medical students to experience medicine in the "real world" outside the halls of academia. Identifying the wants and needs of medical students is critical to providing a successful preceptorship environment. Although a student's wants are unique to the individual physician-in-training, common themes are generally present, and certain needs are common to most medical students.

How are preceptors to understand the wants of individual students? Owing to the diversity of interests among medical students, one can assume little about their expectations. The preceptor would likely find it helpful to ask the student to make a list of personal and professional developmental goals at the beginning of the rotation. The preceptor may be surprised to find goals as diverse as the following examples.

Student 1: obtain experience with flexible sigmoidoscopy and exercise stress testing, learn principles of preventive medicine, learn concepts of the management of common chronic medical conditions such as hypertension and diabetes.

Student 2: learn aspects of women's health, prenatal care, management of menopause, management of common gynecologic complaints, Pap smears, and colposcopy.

Student 3: get experience with management of common acute care problems, including URIs, febrile children, laceration repair, and dermatologic complaints.

The preceptor may find that some medical students want the freedom to see patients independently in order to exercise their history-taking and examination skills, whereas others may simply want to "shadow" the physician and learn by observation. Armed with knowledge of the student's expectations, the preceptor can better tailor the experience to meet the needs of the student while balancing his or her own teaching and practice styles.

For medical students, one of the most exciting aspects of a community rotation is the opportunity to see in a role model the primary reason many of them went into medicine: the magic of the doctor-patient relationship. Students want to learn and practice effective doctor-patient communication. After demonstrating appropriate professional attitudes and interpersonal skills, the preceptor may then want to allow the student to take the lead during a patient encounter. Afterward, the preceptor and student can work as a team to evaluate the encounter. "What were this patient's concerns? What methods did we (you) use to get the patient to express these concerns fully? What else might we (you) have done to better relate to this patient?"

Students want and need experience in various procedures. Whereas some students eagerly jump at the opportunity to perform office procedures such as sigmoidoscopy or colposcopic biopsy, others may be more reluctant out of fear of failing, and may need some prodding to gain more experience and confidence.

Teaching procedural skills is one of the most common forms of teaching in medicine, beginning even in the anatomy lab. "See one. Do one. Teach one" is the axiom for much of our professional training. When "teaching one" to a medical student, the preceptor must remember that the student's understanding is many levels below that of the teacher, and the student may need simple yet complete step-by-step explanations and instructions.

When performing procedures or demonstrating technical skills, students want and need critical but nonjudgmental feedback. For example, "You seem to be having difficulty with . . ." is preferable to "You aren't doing very well at . . ." Whenever possible, criticism should be in the form of "positive-critical-positive." For example, "You performed the punch biopsy smoothly, and you handled the specimen appropriately (positive). You appear to have difficulty suturing the defect. You need to . . . (critical)." Then, after the student attempts to incorporate the feedback and performs the task, the preceptor should provide appropriate positive reinforcement.

Although the "wants" of medical students on rotations with community preceptors are unique to the individual, the "needs" are more easily generalized. Students need timely, specific feedback and assessment of their knowledge and skills, coupled with appropriate instruction to improve their knowledge and skills.

The assessment of a student's knowledge is best done in a nonthreatening way. Students respond much more positively to preceptors whom they perceive as a colleague wanting to assist them in their maturation as a physician, as opposed to the role of mere critic and judge. "Pimping," or asking a series of increasingly arcane questions until the student is stumped, is potentially alienating and an ineffective way to assess the student's knowledge. Questions should be clinically relevant, and their scope can address merely the student's fund of knowledge, or preferably the student's ability to analyze and synthesize data.

As the preceptor identifies areas of strength and weakness in a student, the preceptor can serve as a guide for focused instruction. "Thinking out loud" about a patient's medical problems is an effective and nonthreatening way to communicate clinical information to students. In addition to evidence-based medicine, students appreciate learning from the preceptor's clinical experience with particular problems, describing how past approaches have and have not worked. This not only reinforces the idea of medicine as art, but also plants the seed in the students' minds that they, too, will have trials and errors and therapeutic failures, but these in themselves do not make them bad physicians.

Finally, what medical students need and want most is your time. In the fifth century B.C., Hippocrates recognized the necessity of sacrificing time to teach physicians-in-training. Doctors for centuries have taken the Oath of Hippocrates, which compels physicians "to teach [medical students] this art if they so desire without fee or written promise . . . [these] disciples who have enrolled themselves and have agreed to the rules of the profession." (From *Hippocrates*, "Epidemics I," translated by W. H. S. Jones in the Loeb Classical Library, Cambridge: Harvard University Press, 1923.)

Quality instruction of medical students in a community setting carries the price of the preceptor's time. The actual cost of this sacrifice and ways to minimize it are addressed elsewhere in this book. However, the fact remains that the preceptor's time is one of the most prized gifts that can be given to a student physician. The highest ratings given by medical students to community preceptors are almost always accompanied by comments such as, "He would sit down with me and go over a patient's disease and management," and "She loved to explain things to me."

The community physician preceptor has an exciting opportunity to serve as a role model for medical students and to provide the most meaningful contribution to the profession of medicine. To be successful in this venture, the preceptor must identify the wants and needs of the individual student and commit the time necessary for appropriate instruction. The preceptor will find that this enjoyable sacrifice carries rewards beyond any earthly measure.

■ 5

Learning Needs
of Medical Students

Mary Ann Manners, M.S.P.H.

Key Points
- Medical students have different learning needs at different stages of their medical education.
- Knowledge of these needs can improve your teaching.

Other chapters in this book address what students want and what institutions expect from preceptors. Another component of the preceptorship experience is what the students *need* from preceptors. Learning is a cumulative process, and community physicians are uniquely positioned to aid medical students' development in many areas: communication, clinical skills, personal or psychological needs, and selection of a specialty. The challenge is that while some similarities exist, individual student needs vary. In addition, with recent changes in the curricula at many institutions, the breadth of needs has grown wider because preceptors are now working with students from years one through four in medical school. Owing to the shift toward early clinical exposure during the first and second years of medical school, special attention is essential to meet the learning needs of all levels of students.

As a potential preceptor, you must first decide which students you want to teach, based on your personal preferences and your office personnel and patients. There is a time commitment with all groups, but the focus will differ, depending on the educational level of the students. For example, in most schools first-year students are not yet ready to deliver babies. Recently, however, we had a student excitedly report that during the summer block rotation after his first year, he was asked to actually deliver the newborn during the birth he thought he was just observing. While we hope this was a reflection of the unusually advanced skills and maturity of this particular student, it is more likely that the preceptor was so accustomed to third- and fourth-year students that he forgot to adjust his expectations when the practice started working with first- and second-year students. Your local medical college can help you decide which level of student fits best with your practice by explaining the current curriculum and the experience of students at each level.

Recognizing that curricula differ from institution to institution, the following are some guidelines in addressing the developmental needs of medical students who may work in your practice. There is no substitute for spending time talking with students to assess their knowledge, experience, and maturity. As mentioned in Chapter 10 on orientation, taking time to discuss the students' experiences, their perceived strengths and weaknesses, and what they wish to achieve will enable you to tailor your approach to each student. However, as a preceptor, you have insight about some student needs about which they themselves may be unaware (Whitman and Schwenk, 1995).

Guidelines for Addressing Student Needs

M1–M2 Students

In Chapter 18, Jonas and Bauer categorize first- and second-year students as *neophytes*, evolving to an *apprentice* toward the end of the second year. To meet the developmental needs for this preclinical level, preceptors need to provide:

1. Role models who apply the skills the students are learning early in the curriculum, such as:
   - active listening and interviewing skills (history of present illness, past medical history, family history, social history)
   - holistic patient care and continuity of care with individuals and families
   - practicing the "art" of medicine, including the following communication skills:
     - making patients comfortable about uncomfortable topics
     - phrasing questions to get the best responses
     - taking a complete history on a new patient versus a focused history
     - educating patients and families
     - drawing out quiet or shy patients
     - interacting with more than one person in the room (Wilkerson, Armstrong, and Lesky, 1990)

2. Mentors, who are the next step beyond role model. Take time to sit and talk with students to help them:
   - make the mental adjustment to becoming a physician
   - assess things they enjoy in medicine and identify what scares them
   - determine which areas they might like to pursue
   - identify strategies to have an outside family life
   - develop methods for grappling with ethical issues
   - accept formative feedback, or coaching hints to improve current performance (covered in Chapter 15)

   It is easy to forget the huge psychological transition that occurs during the first years of medical school. Students may find it difficult to discuss these topics in the medical school setting for fear of being judged, saying something not popular, or being perceived as weak. The students really need a safe arena to pursue their personal reactions, and begin the process of developing self-awareness related to medicine.

3. Encouragement that the students can master the overwhelming mass of material, and actually use it, and that they recognize the importance of acknowledging their weaknesses. Luckily, seeing actual patients with a specific problem and disease entity encourages the application of book knowledge and problem solving. It also makes the material easier to learn and retain and reinforces student motivation. Students need to gradually move from only observing the preceptor to doing some activities on their own and comparing each. Establishing a supportive environment in which gaps in knowledge and mistakes are considered a part of learning will allow students to admit weaknesses rather than cover them up.

4. Application of the rudimentary skills they have learned in the following areas:
   - Interviewing, listening, getting the patient's perspective. Students interview patients, then observe the preceptor conduct the interview and compare styles and results. Encourage students to have patients tell them what it's like to have DM, cancer, a child with a birth defect, turn 65, lose a spouse—*to see and feel* the diseases from the patient's perspective, rather than from textbook descriptions. Community physicians quickly learn who the good "teachers" are among their patient population, and the patients usually enjoy their teaching role.
   - Basic physical exam skills. Students take vital signs and eye, ear, throat, heart, and lung exams as they learn them, reinforcing the normals initially, then

see if they can pick up abnormalities. Great opportunities exist in community offices for demonstrating ranges of normal to ranges of abnormal. Some preceptors add structure to the students' experience, such as having a student look at every patient's eyes on a specific day—in addition to whatever other problem a patient may have. After each patient, or at the end of the day, the students can discuss their findings. The next day the preceptor chooses another organ or system to check, depending on what students are learning in their curriculum, or what patients are scheduled.

- They may brainstorm differential diagnoses, making elementary recommendations (for M2s) for simple, one-problem cases.
- Taking a thorough history, practicing physician examination skills, and writing up a case, without worrying yet about efficient use of time, or where to cut corners.

5. Knowledge of office routine:
   - triage and handling patient phone calls
   - office lab versus independent lab
   - roles of other office personnel
   - learning from the nursing staff and other practical hints
   - charting, writing prescriptions

6. Experiencing a physician's lifestyle:
   - how to set aside family time
   - balancing professional and personal activities
   - variety of roles in the community (i.e., volunteer work for schools or church)

7. Aspects of community health:
   - farming health issues
   - local industry problems
   - school and sports health involvement

M3–M4 Students

Jones and Bauer might categorize third- and fourth-year students as *early apprentices*, moving toward the *master* level by the end of the fourth year. To meet the developmental needs for the clinical years, preceptors should provide:

1. Role models who are knowledgeable about and practice current medicine, along with the "gold standard" traditional practices, including:
   - developing the most effective communication techniques, along with personal style
   - remaining current with the literature
   - picking and choosing from each new treatment or drug that comes along

2. Mentors willing to share personal experiences and coping techniques for situations the students may soon encounter, such as:
   - the death of a patient
   - making mistakes
   - handling patients who are not particularly likeable
   - dealing with patient situations the student might oppose, such as abortion or euthanasia
   - formative feedback, suggestions to reinforce or improve current performance (covered more thoroughly in Chapter 15)

   Just being willing to discuss sensitive issues sends a powerful message that these are difficult situations, and it is normal to wrestle with them.

3. More experience in physical exams, and in building skills and confidence in techniques such as:
   - suturing
   - casting
   - pelvic and prostate exams
   - delivering babies

All activities should be appropriate for the student's educational level and experience.

4. Handling complicated cases and challenging situations, including:
   - patients with multiple problems
   - recognizing normal and abnormal findings
   - giving bad news to patients and families
   - drug and alcohol screening interviews
   - angry, manipulative, or seductive patients
   - personality disorders

   Initially students should observe interactions, then take a more active role in patient interaction. For more information on this topic, see Young et al. (1998).

5. Office management and practice activities such as:
   - interactions with other professionals and making referrals
   - use of the health care team in practice
   - call schedules and coverage
   - practical integration of preventive medicine and occupational medicine
   - patient education and resources, brochures, videotapes, etc.
   - office, hospital, nursing home time proportions
   - constraints of insurance, managed care, Medicare and Medicaid, effects on continuity
   - *beginning* to think of time management

6. Pursuing specialty preferences, with open discussion of the following:
   - aspects of practice that are appealing and those that are not
   - pluses and minuses of different specialities
   - questions to ask when choosing a specialty or looking at residencies

- rewards and frustrations of the preceptor's life or practice
- small private practice, multispecialty practices, rural vs. urban, etc.

7. Using local resources, identifying agencies; team approach, interacting with community organizations, schools, volunteer agencies.

Medical school is an immense, multifaceted, sometimes overwhelming process for our students. Community preceptors have the unique potential for helping the students put all the pieces together, gain self-confidence and skills, start to look at specialties, and begin the psychological adjustments that turn students into physicians. With thought and preparation put into guiding the students' experiences in your office, watching the students grow will be a powerful and rewarding experience.

References

Whitman, N., and Schwenk, T. 1995. *Preceptors as Teachers: A Guide to Clinical Teaching*, 2d ed. University of Utah School of Medicine, Salt Lake City, Utah.

Wilkerson, L., Armstrong, E., and Lesky, L. 1990. Faculty development for ambulatory teaching. *Journal of General Internal Medicine* 5:S44–S53.

Young, B. L., Graham, J., Shipengrover, R. P., and James, P.A. 1998. Components of learning in ambulatory settings: a qualitative analysis. *Academic Medicine* 73 (10) (Suppl.): S60–63.

▪ 6

The Teaching Moment

Neal Whitman, Ed.D., and Michael K. Magill, M.D.

Key Points
- ▪ Teaching moments occur both predictably and at random during preceptorships.
- ▪ Information learned during teaching moments is retained for a long time.
- ▪ Learning during teaching moments can be optimized.

The purpose of this chapter is to help you handle one special aspect of human relations in the teaching-learning process: how to optimize the "teaching moment" when a special event has occurred in your practice. In a study at the University of Iowa, medical students were asked, "What unique learning experiences did you have on your family medicine preceptorship as compared to all other rotations to date during your third year?" (Gjerde, Levy, and Xakellis, 1998). Perhaps the most dramatic response was "Actually delivered a baby; didn't get to on Ob/Gyn rotation."

Other experiences, perhaps less dramatic, were nevertheless as important. For example, one student commented, "It was one of the first opportunities to feel like a physician." Gjerde and colleagues concluded, "The family medicine preceptorship was not merely a repeat of what is experienced on the traditional major rotations." To help you develop your skills as a preceptor, this chapter offers teaching strategies to optimize both planned and unplanned learning events.

Planned Events: The Teacher's Use of the Learning Cycle

Sometimes you can anticipate a teaching moment. For example, you have been following the pregnancy of one of your regular patients and the estimated birth date coincides with a student's rotation in your office. Viewing learning as a cycle helps optimize this teaching moment. This view was pioneered by Kolb, who saw learning as a four-stage circular process in which "concrete experience" (having an experience) is followed by "reflection and observation" (reviewing the experience). This leads to "abstract conceptualization" (thinking about and drawing conclusions from the experience). The implications of this experience are then tested in "active experimentation," which provides new experiences subject to review, conceptualization, and more experimentation (Kolb, 1985).

■ *Concrete experience*: To help the student get involved in the experience, you could let the student know that in addition to assisting you in the delivery, he or she will participate in the patient's last prenatal visit. The student should plan during that visit to ask the patient about her expectations and hopes for the delivery.

■ *Reflection and observation*: To help the student think about and reflect on the experience, you could ask the student to explore the patient's perception during the delivery and to interview her before leaving the hospital to determine her assessment of the experience.

■ *Abstract conceptualization*: To help the student generate some lessons, you could instruct the student to develop and discuss with you a model to explain the patient's expectations, hopes, and experience.

■ *Active experimentation*: To help the student test and revise those lessons, you could encourage the student to interview other women. Also, alert the student to the process of learning how patients view all aspects of medical care—a reflection that should continue through medical school and resident training and into medical practice.

Unplanned Events: The Teacher's Use of Witnessing

Sometimes you cannot anticipate a teaching moment; for example, a patient's unexpected death may occur during a student's rotation in your office. Witnessing can optimize this teaching moment. Witnessing is a tool that requires a learner to (1) take a deep breath, (2) step outside himself or herself, (3) take note and observe, and (4) ask "Who am I?" "Why am I here?" and "What am I doing?"

For example, imagine that you perform a cesarean section on a neighbor who lives two doors down the street from you. She develops unavoidable complications and dies four hours later. Understandably, you are now focused on your feelings and the family's needs, *not* the student's feelings and needs. Be aware of *that*, letting the student know that nevertheless he or she should stay by your side.

Ask the student to take note of everything that happens and observe what transpires (e.g., the student may see you sob when you splash cold water on your face before meeting with the family to tell them the bad news). The student should remain with you when you meet the family and talk with colleagues, in person or on the phone.

When you feel ready, perhaps 48 or 72 hours later, meet alone with the student and exchange your own witnessing of this event. And remember: You are only human; you do not have to be perfect.

Viewing learning as a cycle for planned events and using the tool of witnessing for unplanned events can optimize teaching moments. Since these methods depend on two-way interaction, this chapter can be seen as complementary to Chapter 11 on learning contracts.

References

Gjerde, C. L., Levy, B. T., and Xakellis, G. C., Jr. 1998. Unique learning contributions of a family medicine preceptorship. *Family Medicine* 30:410–16.

Kolb, D. A. 1985. *Learning Style Inventory*. Boston: McBer and Co.

■ III

Clinical Teaching

▪ 7

Learning during the Preceptorship

Steven L. Lawrence, M.D., and David Olson, M.D.

Key Points
- Staff and patient support for the preceptorship are critical elements for success.
- Successful teachers actively involve learners, promote learner autonomy, demonstrate patient care skills, and provide feedback.
- Effective preceptors are also role models and mentors.

As medical student education moves out of the academic health science center, there are increased opportunities for community physicians to become involved in education. While a number of community physicians have long been involved in medical student education, many are new to this role. This chapter explores factors that promote student learning during the preceptorship.

When you choose to begin precepting students, it is extremely important to elicit the support of your staff and patients. Involvement of your staff in your teaching endeavor enhances the learning environment for the student, as explained later. A brief information handout given to your patients at the time they register can set the stage for their acceptance of medical students. Reassure your patients that they will be seen by you and that you view the presence of students as "value added" for the patient. Students generally spend more time with patients, discussing their medical needs, something most patients appreciate. Let them know they can request *not* to be seen by a student, if they so desire.

What can you do to provide an office experience that facilitates learning for your medical students? Research has identified characteristics of effective clinical teachers that affect overall teaching effectiveness. A University of Washington medical school survey (Irby et al., 1991) identified the most important characteristics for ambulatory teachers: They actively involve the learners, promote learner autonomy, and demonstrate patient care skills. Clinic environment variables, such as structured time for teaching, space for teaching, clinical case mix, workload, or organization of the clinic were deemed less important.

How are these characteristics translated into office behavior? At the student's first visit to your office, spend a few minutes learning about the student as a person and what they hope to learn out of this clinical rotation. Introduce them to staff and colleagues. Show them around the clinic and exam rooms where you will be seeing patients. Explain to them that you will see patients together until the student feels comfortable and develops the skills to see patients on his or her own. Some practices have the student become a "patient" the first day, having the nurse or office manager take them through registration, insurance verification, and into the exam room. During this time, the student meets the office team and learns about their roles. This process effectively orients the learner to their learning environment and positively involves your staff.

Encourage the student to have direct patient contact. Initially, let them observe a few of your patient encounters. After a couple of days, encourage the student's learning autonomy by having them see the patient first and take the patient's history, then have them present the history to you. You can then see the patient together, take the history, do the pertinent exam, and model appropriate assessment and medical decision-making. After leaving the exam room, discuss and compare the student's history with your own. After a few days, ask the student to not only take the appropriate history but also a focused physical exam. The student now presents both history and the pertinent physical findings to you. Sometimes you can discuss a possible assessment and plan before going in and seeing the patient together, or you may wait until you have taken the history and completed the exam. Both approaches actively involve the learner and demonstrate patient care skills. As the student's skills progress, provide increasing autonomy within the boundaries of sound medical practice.

As the rotation proceeds, students want to know how they are progressing, even though they may not ask. It is helpful to provide continuing feedback while making a point of giving the student constructive comments at the midpoint and end of the rotation. It is important that the preceptor assist students in their professional growth by providing constructive feedback. Constructive feedback focuses on timely, helpful correction of problems observed in professional knowledge, skills, behaviors, and attitudes. For example, if you saw that your student was not making adequate eye contact with a patient during an interview, you might discuss this observation immediately after the encounter. Explain why it is desirable to increase eye contact with patients and demonstrate that behavior for the student.

Precepting goes beyond just teaching these basic medical skills. We are role models who advise, who guide, and who mentor. Mentoring has a long history in the professions. The father of medicine, Hippocrates, encouraged doctors to share their wisdom with younger physicians. He encouraged older doctors to guide and welcome new student doctors. The mentor serves as a role model, facilitator, and teacher for junior physicians. The mentor introduces the student to the customs and mores of the field of medicine and to the social aspect of being a doctor. He or she links the practice of medicine to the community and the rich history of what it means to be a doctor. Preceptorships give you, the experienced clinician, a tremendous opportunity to allow the student insights into the meaning of being a doctor.

Even if we provide our enthusiasm and mentorship, how do we know that students learn during the preceptorship? Recent research demonstrated that students in a family medicine preceptorship experienced "substantial learning and reinforcement," and acquired skills that were unique to the ambulatory setting (e.g., management of acute sprains and strains, low-back pain, sinusitis, strep throat, acute bronchitis, and osteoarthritis) (Gjerde, Levy, and Xakellis, 1998). Our own research has shown that students highly value their time alone with patients to practice their skill in taking histories and performing physicals, enhancing their development of doctor-patient relationships, and improving their clinical decision-making. They also highly value observing their preceptors as they interact with patients, demonstrate examination techniques, and formulate diagnoses and management plans (Lawrence, Lindemann, and Gottlieb, 1999).

What do you, the preceptor, derive from this experience? A study by Grayson et al. (1998) demonstrated that 82 percent of preceptors increased their enjoyment of the practice of medicine. Preceptors reported spending more time reviewing clinical medicine and keeping up with the literature while patients' perception of their status improved. In spite of the costs (a reported decrease in the number of patients seen), the authors concluded that clinicians derive net benefits from providing primary care preceptorships to medical students.

In summary, learning during the preceptorship appears to depend heavily on the preceptor's actively involving the learner in the process, encouraging the learner's autonomy, establishing rapport with the learner, and providing timely, constructive feedback.

References

Gjerde, C. L., Levy, B. T., and Xakellis, G. C., Jr. 1998. Unique learning contributions of a family medicine preceptorship. *Family Medicine* 30:410–16.

Grayson, M., Klein, M., Lugo, J., and Visintainer, P. 1998. Benefits and cost to community-based physicians teaching primary care to medical students. *Journal of General Internal Medicine* 13:485–88.

Irby, D., Ramsey, P. G., Gillmore, G. M., and Schaad, D. 1991. Characteristics of effective clinical teachers of ambulatory care medicine. *Academic Medicine* 66:51–55.

Lawrence, S. L., Lindemann, J. C., and Gottlieb, M. 1999. What students value: learning outcomes in a required third-year ambulatory primary care clerkship. *Academic Medicine* 74(6): 715–17.

8

Being a Role Model

Rick E. Ricer, M.D.

Key Points

- All preceptors are role models; in fact, community physicians may be the most powerful role models for students.
- Qualifications of a good role model include charisma, leadership, competence, compassion, honesty, consistency, and a strong work ethic.
- Mentors share values, provide emotional support, and facilitate career development.

Role models are persons whose behaviors, personal styles, and specific attributes are emulated by others. As a community physician, you are a role model for your patients, students, residents, neighbors, colleagues, and children. Being a role model is a passive process and can be positive or negative. You can be a role model with regard to careers, attitudes, values, and behaviors.

Most people have more than one role model—individuals who have traits with which they identify or which they want to learn or imitate. People have a tendency to emulate role models perceived to be like themselves. Role models may range from personal friends to well-known figures such as sports stars. You are probably unaware that you are a role model to many people. Most of us can recall many people in our lives that we have used as role models.

For medical students, the practicing community physician is usually a very positive role model, an example, or even an ideal after which they can pattern their own behavior. As a community preceptor, you may be the first role model your students encounter who is not a university physician. Therefore, your interactions may be critical to their development. Your actions, behaviors, gestures, phrases, and demeanor while interacting with patients, families, and staff will be observed and may be emulated by your students. You should take care to provide a model of behavior you would be proud to have students adopt.

"Role modeling" is just one of the common terms used to describe the interactions that community physicians may have with medical students. Terms can be confusing and overlapping, especially since one community physician may fill various roles concurrently or at different times in a student's life.

"Preceptor," "mentor," and "counselor" are terms that can be confused with "role model." Much of this book is devoted to precepting. Most simply, a preceptor is a clinical teacher. The teaching is usually done outside the classroom, in the office and sometimes the hospital, and is typically a one-on-one tutorial relationship. The preceptorial experience may be part of a formal course, with the preceptor evaluating the performance of the student.

A counselor may do many things, but most often counselors are active listeners and advisors. Although the term "counseling" is not meant to imply the provision of psychotherapy, counselors may advise students on what courses to take, how to deal with personal and professional problems, and how to interact with patients, and they may provide advice on careers.

Mentoring often connotes a deeper relationship that may encompass the former roles and terms. A mentor is more of a coach or trusted friend. Mentoring is a personal process that combines role modeling, apprenticeship, counseling, and nurturing. One definition of mentorship is an intense, multifaceted process in which an experienced individual serves as teacher, sponsor, and advisor to a student; provides for the personal growth of the student; and derives personal growth from the process (Ricer, Fox, and Miller, 1995). This is usually a long-term relationship that must develop over time. Role models are not necessarily mentors, but mentors always serve as role models. Mentors do not formally evaluate the mentee. Mentors share values, provide emotional support, facilitate access to career development, and give career counseling. They also protect, challenge, confirm, accept, befriend, and encourage the mentee (Shapiro, Hasseltine, and Rowe, 1978). Mentors are developers of talent and serve as confidants for the mentee.

The qualities of a good role model, preceptor, mentor, or counselor are exactly the same qualities possessed by a community physician. Charisma, leadership, motivation, inspiration, competence, compassion and empathy, honesty, consistency, and a strong work ethic are all qualities most community physicians possess.

Positive exposure to practicing community physicians is critical to a successful medical school or residency program. Many medical schools could not fulfill their mission without the assistance of practicing community physicians. Your efforts and involvement with the students will be very rewarding and greatly appreciated.

References

Ricer, R. E., Fox, B. C., and Miller, K. E. 1995. Mentoring for medical students interested in family practice. *Family Medicine* 27(6):360–65.

Shapiro, E. C., Hasseltine, F. P., and Rowe, M. P. 1978. Moving up: role models, mentors and the "patron system." *Sloan Management Review* 19(3):51–58.

9

Integrating the Student
into the Practice

Walter L. Larimore, M.D.

Key Points

Students can be smoothly integrated into your practice by following these principles:
- Negotiate expectations and goals.
- Orient the student.
- Provide regular feedback.
- Encourage the student to teach and to do self-directed learning.
- Organize your practice for teaching.

It is possible to learn how to successfully integrate a student into a busy private practice; however, becoming a successful and satisfied preceptor will require that you learn to include others in the teaching process. Said another way, efficient and effective precepting of students means integrating them into your office by maximizing your own time and the efforts of your team. In my practice, I am not the only preceptor for the students who visit—my family, my partners, my practice employees, and my colleagues in the community all help educate the student.

This type of precepting requires preparation and planning by the doctor and his or her staff before the first student ever arrives. It involves coming up with a strategy and then orchestrating your game plan with aplomb. This approach allows us to provide an immersion experience for the students who come to our practice. We do not just sprinkle them "in the faith," we immerse them! They live, wake, eat, sleep, practice, attend rounds, deliver care, home visit, operate, work, and play in and with the entire community.

Most of my students came believing they would "rather see a sermon than hear one any day." They often depart saying, "I'd rather be a sermon than see one any day." What could you do to more fully integrate the students whom you have the honor of mentoring in your practice? Here are a few suggestions for procedures that have helped us.

Intake Interview and Negotiation

In my practice, intake interview and negotiation are done in a meeting that includes one doctor, one nurse, and one front-office staff member, each of whom has the responsibility to let the others in their department know the results of the meeting. During this meeting, I seek to establish a learning contract (see Chapter 11) and a teaching contract and to set goals and objectives (see Chapter 12). This meeting is extremely important. Students are much more likely to perform effectively and learn efficiently when they know what we expect of them and when we know what they expect of us. Here is what we do:

■ Find out what they think they know and what they think they want. Obtaining this information requires us to ask a number of questions. With what problems and clinical areas do they feel comfortable? With what subjects, what type of patients, what procedures have they had experience? Where are they in their training? How much clinical experience have they had? What are their career goals (see Chapter 4)? If they do not plan to become family physicians, I do not see it as my role to "convert" them, and I tell them this. But I let them know that learning how a family physician thinks and why we do what we do will help them if they choose a specialty where referrals from family physicians are important. In other words, I let them know that this rotation will make them a much more successful consultant than their classmates.

- Find out what and how they want to learn. Inquire about their preferred learning style. Do they understand active versus passive learning? Do they prefer to shadow you or go solo (see patients alone first)? Do they want to spend all of their time with patients or do they want some reading and study time? Do they want to stay with one doctor the whole time, or do they want a variety of preceptors? What do they want to learn when they are with you? What do they want to accomplish? Negotiate a learning contract (see Chapter 11).

- Find out what they'll do. Just how much do they want to be part of both the practice's life and your personal and community life? What office hours and night hours do they want to work? What about weekends? Let them know your minimum expectations. Negotiate a schedule.

- Let them know their options for educational experiences in your network of consultants and colleagues. The students that visit my practice are encouraged to visit a variety of other health care providers in the community during their stay with us. They can visit with other family physicians who have different types of practices: an osteopathic family physician, a family physician specializing in occupational health or sports medicine. They have in-hospital opportunities (ER or surgery or obstetrics with family physicians). I like them to spend at least a half day with a home health department director (who is a family physician). They can also travel to a nearby city to spend some time in medical administration (with a family physician HMO

director) or space medicine (with one of the family
physician astronauts). In addition, we have a number
of "family practice-friendly" consultants who can take
the student for a half day if the student wants more
intensive exposure to a particular procedure or
specialty (see Chapter 21).

■ Let the student know all your expectations and
weaknesses. This list may change with time. Your
nurse can help with the list of your weaknesses. It is
helpful to discuss this and then give it to the student
in a written form. Communicate what you plan to
teach and what you propose to accomplish while they
are there.

■ Let them know who will evaluate them, how they will
be evaluated, and when their evaluation will be
completed (see Chapter 16).

Orientation

Orientation is usually done by my staff. I want the student to quickly become comfortable in our practice environment. I want the students to be familiar with (a) the
clinical area and clinical protocols and procedures (explained by the nursing staff); (b) office equipment, forms,
phones (explained by the administrative staff); (c) what it
is like to be a patient and the admission and treatment
routine (a nurse actually has them call for an appointment and then go through an entire visit as a patient);
(d) the town (a tour is given by a local realtor or a spouse);
(e) the hospital (a tour is given by the hospital administrator; see Chapter 28); and (f) where they will stay (see
Chapter 10).

Daily Feedback

Daily coaching is critical. It is important that feedback
goes both ways, from student to teacher and vice versa. I

always seek feedback and criticism first; then I give positive feedback freely, and finally I discuss what needs improvement. I try to provide corrective feedback that is timely, specific, and descriptive (how to improve and make things easier and tricks of the trade) (see Chapter 15).

Teach the Student to Teach and to Do Self-Directed Learning

I ask the student to teach at a conference or lunch meeting at least once while they are at our practice. Ask the doctors and nurses to attend (buying lunch guarantees a crowd). Help your student become an expert in one subject while he or she is with you. If you choose a topic in which you need to brush up, both you and the student can gain enormously from the student's teaching. Students seem to retain information more effectively when they teach.

During the day, give them time to read and do Internet or journal searches. Allow them time for reflection, reading, and self-directed learning. If a student sees an interesting case and wants to stop to read about it, they can learn while I go on seeing patients.

Delegate Responsibility

Give the student some responsibility during the clinical hours. Let them preround on your hospital patients before rounding with you. Assign particular patients or cases to the student. Provide opportunities for active involvement by the student. Teach the student how to teach patients and then let the student do patient education. Of course, you need to tailor these assignments to the student's level of expertise and experience.

Also delegate teaching responsibility to your staff. Early in their visit, students spend a half day with our lab and

X-ray staff and our appointment and reception staff. The students are often surprised at how much they learn about medicine, people, the practice, and the community. Allow other health care providers in your community to help you with the teaching. It makes a better experience for the student and decreases the demands on your time.

Exit Interview and Negotiation

I have all my staff complete our anonymous evaluation tool about the student. This tool allows staff to share observations about the student's personal characteristics and traits (e.g., timeliness, neatness, and compassion). At a formal "sit-down" session, I try to share these observations: (a) strengths (personal and professional) that the staff and I observed and (b) blind spots or weaknesses that we observed that need to be improved or corrected. Most important, I share strategies for strengthening both strong and weak areas (see Chapter 16).

Practice and Patient Flow Changes

Our practice has learned that there are a number of daily activities that help us integrate students more easily:

(a) Nurses talk at their morning meeting about cases that are scheduled that day. Which cases would be good for the student and which may not be appropriate?

(b) The doctor that is working with the student needs to arrive a bit early to organize his or her day and meet with the student.

(c) The doctor reviews the day's schedule with nurse and student before seeing patients.

(d) The doctor who is with the student sets aside extra time during each half day (one or two 15-minute slots) for talking, teaching, and catch-up.

(e) Every patient is not seen by every student and every patient is given the option of choosing whether the student sees them. If possible, this is done when the appointment is made; it is confirmed when the patient checks in and is reconfirmed by the nurse.

(f) Have the student carry a pad for writing down questions that can be discussed after patient hours. Encourage the student to ask questions, although many can be discussed at a later time. Some of my sweetest memories of teaching come from times spent with students after hours or while in the car traveling from one location to another. Instead of answering questions, try turning around a student's query. Ask them what they think. What would they do? Then share what you might do.

(g) Aim to teach one "take-home point" per half day of clinical time. Look for teachable moments. Often these "nuggets" are remembered for a lifetime, long after textbook lessons have been forgotten.

We don't teach our students about the science of family practice or what it is; we show them what family physicians are, and what they do, and why they do what they do. My family, staff, church, and community all participate in both the teaching and the learning. We are integrated into the student's life as the student is integrated into ours. That seems to be what the students want the most and it seems to be what we enjoy the most. Maybe that's why so many come back to visit, even years and years after graduation. Maybe that's why we have so many Christmas cards from them. Maybe that's why we have so many wonderful and special memories of incredible relationships that were started, built, continued, and cherished through a simple preceptorship that integrates a doctor-to-be with a community and a community with a doctor-to-be.

■ 10

Orienting Medical Students

David J. Steele, Ph.D.

Key Points
- ■ A formal orientation process enhances teaching and learning during the preceptorship.
- ■ Much of the orientation information can be given to the student via written materials.

Orientation is an important aspect of the teaching and learning transaction in the ambulatory care setting, but it is one that is all too often short changed. Potentially powerful messages are sent to the learner by the way the preceptor manages the introduction of the student into the practice. This introduction can set the tone for the entire experience. Done properly, an orientation can significantly reduce student anxiety and pave the way for an enhanced learning experience. Unfortunately, many preceptors do not provide such an orientation. A few moments spent orienting the student can save the preceptor time and allow students to concentrate on learning activities. The items that should be included in an orientation are summarized in Table 10.1. Much of this information can be sent to the student in written form prior to the rotation.

A portion of the student's orientation can be delegated to a nurse, office manager, or other knowledgeable member of the support staff. The staff can show the student

This chapter is based on work previously published in *Family Medicine* 29(9):614–15.

Table 10.1. ■ Orientation topics

Topic to Be Discussed with Student	Discussion Points
Staff	Names, titles, roles, special interest, and competencies
The community and the clinic	Location (address, map, phone numbers)
	Brief description of the demographics of the community
	Demographic characteristics of the patient population served by the practice
	Special resources
	Laboratory
	Library
	Other specialty and subspecialty practices in the community
Hospital, nursing home, satellite facilities, pharmacies	Emergency department and after-hours activities
Office routine	Office hours, scheduling procedures, and patterns
	Preceptor schedule (e.g., clinic hours, rounds, call schedule, nursing home visits)
	Medical records
	Practice guidelines, protocols employed in practice
	Prescribing
	Recording information
	Countersigning by preceptor
	Supervision of student

Table 10.1. ■ Orientation topics *(continued)*

Topic to Be Discussed with Student	Discussion Points
"Administrative" expectations	Student hours and schedule, call schedule
	Expected role in patient care
	Dress code
	Contact persons for questions, problem solving
	Room and board
Teaching and learning expectations	Student background and experience
	Student learning goals and interests
	Program expectations
	Preceptor's special skills, interest, and teaching and learning expectations
	Scheduled time for feedback, midcourse corrections, and debriefing

around the office, describe standard procedures for registering and moving patients through the clinic, review charting procedures, and explain the practice routine.

Other issues are best approached by the preceptor through one-on-one conversations with the learner and cannot be delegated. This discussion may include issues such as the student's schedule, clinical activities, and dress code. The mutual sharing of teaching and learning expectations is one of the most critical components of the orientation process. Spending a few minutes with students at the beginning of their rotations to learn about their background, interests, and goals provides information that is crucial for making informed decisions about how to organize the learning experience.

Because many academic health centers are providing early patient contact, it is important to assess the student's knowledge, experience, and learning expectations. It makes little sense to quiz an inexperienced first-year student about differential diagnosis and treatment recommendations when the student's goal is to observe and practice medical interviews. On the other hand, students late in their third year are likely to grow weary of "shadowing" and will gain more from independent, hands-on patient care experiences. Agreement about goals and expectations sets the stage for student feedback and assessment. A discussion of when and how feedback will be provided should be included in the orientation.

The initial orientation need not be lengthy. Many preceptors accomplish their orientation in less than 30 minutes, particularly when the students have received written materials in advance. A scheduled, explicit discussion of goals and expectations helps create a positive learning climate and demonstrates concern for the student.

▪ 11

Learning Contracts

Michael K. Magill, M.D., and Neal Whitman, Ed.D.

Key Points

- ▪ Learning contracts facilitate teaching and learning during the preceptorship.
- ▪ Establishing a learning contract takes very little time.
- ▪ Preceptors have the skills necessary to establish a learning contract with their students.

Teaching adults is more effective and satisfying to both the teacher and learner if they agree on *what* is to be taught and learned and *how* it will be taught and learned. A learning contract is an agreement between a teacher and learner on what is to be learned and how it will be learned. In clinical teaching, it may be (and usually is) informal and personal between a specific teacher and specific learner. The agreement may be implicit rather than explicit. However, it is almost always better to make the contract explicit, open, and negotiated at the beginning of a new relationship between a preceptor and student. The contract should be renegotiated periodically and informally throughout the precepting relationship.

Knowing a student's learning needs will help focus the content, the "what," of the student's initial learning in the medical office. For example, imagine a student with little medical background preparing for his or her first preceptorship experience. Before a student can function seeing patients individually, even to conduct the most rudimentary clinical interview (such as simply asking about the patient's chief complaint), this student may need basic orientation. The student may need to learn the following: how appointments are scheduled, how vital signs are taken, what office nurses do, and what information physicians review before seeing patients.

There are a multitude of strategies (the "how") by which the student can acquire this basic information. For example, the office manager could describe patient flow. The student could then interview and shadow office staff. During this experience, the student could focus on one aspect of the encounter: for example, how each staff member helps evaluate and manage patient problems. The student could observe the office nurse taking chief complaints and recording them in the medical record. The student could then discuss his or her observations with the preceptor prior to independently recording the patient's chief complaints.

Another equally valid approach might be to learn how to take vital signs, document them, and take the chief complaints. The student could then observe the physician taking the patient's history and physical. Using this approach, the student might compare his or her findings with the physician's as a basis for learning a more efficient interviewing style. A focused, brief discussion could orient the student to the roles of office staff. Standard textbooks could supplement this learning and be discussed with the preceptor the following day.

These learning needs (the "what") and strategies (the "how") will differ, depending on the student. Imagine a fourth-year medical student with a prior career as an emergency medical technician. This student may be very comfortable and knowledgeable about the functions of a medical office, the steps in patient evaluation, history taking, and examination. He or she may focus on more complex aspects of clinical decision-making, on acquiring advanced knowledge about common clinical problems, and on improving his or her efficiency in problem-oriented evaluation of patients. The student may be able to independently evaluate patients very competently but would benefit from readings from the original medical literature. This learner will thus focus on different types and levels of knowledge and need a very different style of support and teaching from the preceptor.

How is the preceptor to know what the right content and learning strategy are for a given student? The answer is simple: Remember an old lesson from everyone's childhood, "Stop, look, and listen before you cross the street." Stop and look at the student's nonverbal messages. Confused or blank facial expressions as a student sorts through surgical instruments on a tray may belie the confident assertion that "I've done a lot of these biopsies." Then listen. Listen to the sound of a student's voice as well as his or her words. A student's sparkling eyes and light step may be the only acknowledgment you get for having praised good interviewing skills. Observing these nonverbal cues and behaviors will help you plan future teaching.

Listening, of course, should begin on day one. Only by first listening to a student will you ultimately be heard. At the beginning of the precepting relationship, set aside time to ask about the student's background, prior knowledge, desired learning focus, current stage of training, and preferred approach to learning. This discussion will enable student and preceptor to clarify learning and teaching expectations. Moreover, the formal requirements of the rotation may be difficult to meet in a given office. For example, the student may want to do computerized literature searches, but no computers are available. However, the student's behavior and interests will be driven far more by his or her desired learning than by any external requirements. Knowing these needs and desires is the first step toward negotiating mutually acceptable learning goals and strategies. Some of these goals may originate with the student, some with the medical school, and some with the preceptor.

Once the preceptor and student negotiate a learning plan (a "contract"), they can then implement it, reevaluate as they go, and improve it throughout the precepting relationship. This will help make the relationship one that provides the best possible learning for the student and the most satisfying teaching for the preceptor.

■ **12**

Using Goals and Objectives in Community Rotations

Marian R. Stuart, Ph.D., and
Paula S. Krauser, M.D., M.A.

Key Points
■ Establishing educational goals and objectives during preceptorship facilitates learning by students and evaluation of their performance.
■ Objectives should be:
  S   specific
  M   measurable
  A   attainable
  R   relevant
  T   time-framed

The preceptor for a community rotation plays a crucial but challenging role in training medical students in an ambulatory setting. A considerable body of evidence suggests that having students in the office cuts into the time physicians spend with patients or in leisure activities (Vinson, Paden, and Devera-Sales, 1996; Vinson and Paden, 1994; Garg et al., 1991). Although training medical students may affect productivity negatively, there are many benefits to precepting. Professional growth, increased knowledge, and positive effects on patient satisfaction are some of the rewards of precepting (Usatine et al., 1995).

Students vary greatly in their attitudes toward primary care and have diverse levels of knowledge and skills. Many arrive unprepared for the office setting, having only written long, detailed H&Ps in a hospital setting. Part of the preceptor's responsibility is to evaluate the student's performance at the end of the rotation. Without clear and objective criteria, this can be an exceedingly difficult task. The student's university should provide goals and objectives for the rotation and specify evaluation criteria; however, the physician can enhance the precepting experience by providing the students with site-specific learning goals and objectives (Table 12.1).

Many physicians assume that having the student shadow them or see patients independently will promote learning. Although this is generally true, the experience can be enhanced by setting clear goals and objectives. A goal is a global statement describing the desired outcome of an activity in terms of its effects on the learner. Objectives are specific statements detailing the knowledge, skills, and attitudes that must be acquired to achieve the goal. Goals and objectives help to focus your energies productively, inform the student about what is expected, and ease the evaluation process.

Providing a student with an opportunity to work with a community physician for a period of months is not a goal but an educational strategy. Given that the student completes this requirement, the question becomes: "What changes in knowledge, skills, or attitudes do I hope will

Table 12.1. ■ Sample goal and objectives

Goal	The goal of this clinical experience is to help students appreciate the importance of the doctor-patient relationship.
Objectives	At the end of the rotation, the student will be able to: • describe three behaviors that help enhance the establishment of rapport • demonstrate the ability to conduct a patient-centered interview • give empathic responses during every patient interview

occur as a result of this experience?" The goal of the rotation might be to increase the student's appreciation of the variety of common problems treated effectively by primary care physicians. Another goal might be to increase the student's ability to address problems using a patient-centered interview and a biopsychosocial approach. In other words, a statement of a goal answers the question: "What is it that I hope the student will get from this rotation?" For each goal, several objectives can be developed to detail the particular behaviors that will ensure that the goal has been achieved. These objectives need to be SMART (*s*pecific, *m*easurable, *a*ttainable, *r*elevant, and *t*ime-framed).

Objectives are designed to answer the question: "By the end of the rotation, what specifically do I want the student to know, be able to do, or feel?" By specific, we mean "who should do or know what, how, when, and under what circumstances." Knowledge components are measurable if the student can describe, discuss, list, or explain a designated number of phenomena. In other words, the student must be able to demonstrate acquisition of the knowledge. Skills can be measured, since they can be observed when the student performs them. They can also be measured by the number of trials or how long it takes the student to successfully accomplish a given activity or procedure. Attitudes can be only inferred from the student's willingness to engage in certain activities or make particular commitments. Attainable means that the opportunity to learn exists and it is reasonable to expect the learning to occur during the course of the rotation. Objectives should be relevant to the goal and time-framed (i.e., achievable by the end of the rotation).

The investment of your time spent thinking through the goals and objectives for the rotation will help focus your discussions with the student on critical issues. When you determine your objectives at the beginning, it maximizes the effectiveness of your teaching time and increases your ability to achieve your goals. Sharing the goals and objectives with the student at the start of the rotation has the further benefit of communicating clear expectations about what is to be learned. Finally, the written objectives form the basis for evaluating the student. The evaluation simply becomes a process of checking to see if the objectives have been met (i.e., to what extent the student demonstrates the knowledge, skills, and attitudes that you have specified).

As a community preceptor, you make a significant contribution to the education of future physicians. The discipline of routinely developing goals and objectives for each learner will enhance your teaching effectiveness, the student's appreciation of your specialty, and mutual satisfaction with the experience.

References

Garg, M. L., Boero, J. F., Christiansen, R. G., and Booher, C. G. 1991. Primary care teaching physicians' losses of productivity and revenue at three ambulatory care centers. *Academic Medicine* 66:348–53.

Usatine, R. P., Hodgson, C. S., Marshall, E. T., Whitman, D. W., Slavin, S. J., and Wilkes, M. S. 1995. Reactions of family medicine community preceptors to teaching medical students. *Family Medicine* 27:566–70.

Vinson, D. C., and Paden, C. 1994. The effect of teaching medical students on private practitioners' workloads. *Academic Medicine* 69:237–38.

Vinson, D. C., Paden, C., and Devera-Sales, A. 1996. Impact of medical student teaching on family physicians' use of time. *Journal of Family Practice* 42:243–49.

■ 13

Supervision

Christine C. Matson, M.D., Anne McCarthy, M.D., and Mark Simon, M.D.

Key Points

- The degree of supervision that a student requires depends on both the student's level of education and experience and the characteristics of the preceptor's practice.
- Providing either too much or too little supervision can interfere with a student's learning and place patient outcomes at risk.
- The preceptor should assess the student's learning need for each session and for each patient and provide the appropriate level of supervision based on these needs.
- Students require a balance between support and challenge that varies with each student and with differing levels of education and experience.
- Supervision can be either prospective (anticipatory guidance), concurrent with the student-patient encounter, or retrospective, after the patient encounter (review and reflection). Retrospective supervision is often asynchronous and may be more time efficient than prospective supervision.

Deciding how closely a student needs to be supervised is important for the student's learning needs, the patient's safety, and the medicolegal risk to the preceptor's practice. Providing either too much or too little supervision can adversely affect learning effectiveness and the student's perception of the quality of the experience. The degree of supervision is also a critical determinant of the impact of a student on the preceptor's productivity.

Goals for the preceptorship experience and their impact on level of supervision differ according to the level of the learner. Mentoring is an important aspect at all levels, but especially in the first two years of medical training. Through the mentoring process, students increase their knowledge and skills and learn professional values that are not always included in the written curriculum. They learn to integrate biomedical knowledge from traditional basic medical sciences with the clinical sciences. This integration is required in order to understand human motivation and behavior; the ethical and professional obligations of physicians; and the elements of relationship, patient values, and dealing with uncertainty. Supervision to build skills and the development of a database for evaluating the student assume increasing importance for the more senior student.

The challenge in answering the "How much?" question is to provide the right level of supervision. This varies with the student's experience and learning style, and with characteristics of the preceptor's practice, such as preceptor experience and patients' expectations. Steps to determine the appropriate level include the following:

1. *Determine the student's educational level and comfort level with proposed tasks.* The educational program director should describe students' previous experience (e.g., M3 clerks who had a longitudinal mentorship in M1 and M2). Ask students about their experience in ambulatory or inpatient settings and what level of responsibility they have exercised. Remember that there is a substantial level of variability in student abilities, even at the same educational level.

2. *Assess specific educational needs for particular patient encounters.* If the student has seen patients with similar presentations before and feels comfortable, less supervision may be required than for new situations.

3. *Assess the patients' readiness for student involvement and the potential risk of their medical condition.* Both patients and students feel more comfortable knowing that the patient's physician is ensuring optimal outcomes and avoiding any risk to the patient's safety.

4. *Seek an optimal level of support and challenge.* Most students say they learn best when they have the opportunity to see patients first on their own rather than just "coat-tailing" their preceptors. The need to make a commitment to a patient assessment or a physical finding before review by the preceptor is an effective stimulus for long-term learning. Provide structure for the hesitant or risk-avoidant student, and communicate your expectations for consultation to ensure patient safety for the aggressive or overly confident student.

5. *When the student has interviewed and examined a patient, reassess the student's learning needs.* Asking the student to critique his or her own performance or posing questions such as, "What do you need to know for the next step?" may be a time-efficient way to judge the level of supervision required during a patient encounter.

Table 13.1 describes the types of supervision that can be modified based on the level and competence of the learner and the time available. Concurrent supervision requires that both the patient and the student be present when the supervision occurs; however, some types of pro-

Table 13.1. ■ Types of supervision

Supervision	Example
Prospective	Review curricular objectives for session, if available
	Demonstrate a procedure (e.g., with a drawing) before its performance
	Talk through the approach to a patient in advance
	Ask student to describe next steps
Concurrent	Observe student conducting interview, intervene only when necessary
	Demonstrate physical exam maneuver and ask student to repeat
	Drop in on student and patient for brief periods to sample interview skills
Retrospective	Listen to student's presentation of case history and findings and compare with your own understanding
	Review and discuss student's note in medical record
	Summarize and evaluate patterns of student's interactions with patients at the end of the session
	Discuss student's previous management when a patient returns for follow-up

spective and retrospective supervision allow the time-efficiency of asynchronous teaching. An accurate assessment of the student's learning needs is the best way to plan supervision at the appropriate level so that the student's learning and patient care are optimal.

Teaching and Learning Styles

Dan Benzie, M.D., and Keith Stelter, M.D.

Key Points

■ Knowledge of the student's learning style and the teacher's learning style can improve the teaching and learning experience during the preceptorship.

■ Adapting your teaching style to your student's learning style can optimize the precepting experience.

This chapter focuses on matching teaching styles with students' preferred learning styles. To create a quality learning experience, the community teacher should perform a self-assessment, reach mutual agreement with the student on the intended outcome, and then assess the student's knowledge base and style of learning.

Teacher's Self-Assessment

Reflecting on your own teaching and learning experiences and considering both positive and negative aspects will help you assess your teaching style. It is helpful to think about the physician-patient teaching style that you use each day in the office and to incorporate feedback from experiences with patients, colleagues, or community activities. Defining your own practice interests and style will also influence the methods you choose. There are a number of core attributes exhibited by community clerkship faculty. Excellent clinical teachers have been defined as those who are:

- supportive and respectful to students and patients
- looking for opportunities to provide appropriate role modeling
- enthusiastic about their clinical practice and teaching (Irby, 1995)

A few questions that can be used for self-assessment are:

- How do I interact best with patients?
- What types of techniques do I use to learn new material (e.g., reading, visual, concepts, facts)?
- What do I hope to accomplish for myself and the student by teaching in this period of time?

Review the Intended Outcomes

Your regional medical schools should provide you with understandable and realistic goals and objectives that are specific to the level of your student. Community teachers are encouraged to find out what basic medical principles should be taught in clerkships, to take into account the student's individual goals, and then to determine what outcomes can be expected from the preceptorship. This is further described by Swee (1991).

Whenever possible, try to incorporate an appropriate mix of knowledge, skills, and attitudes into your daily teaching. Specific aspects of knowledge that are helpful relate to common clinical diagnoses seen in a community practice; general principles of prevention and the disease process; and the management of comprehensive long-term health issues or chronic health problems.

Skills that are important to cover in your teaching include patient-physician communication skills (history taking); physical examination skills; problem solving (utilize resources unique to your particular community); and principles of performing and learning procedures common to primary care.

Among the attitudes that are helpful to incorporate in your teaching efforts is professionalism, which is demonstrated through each physician's attitude toward patients, the health care team members, and students. Recognition of the physician as a member of the community and a role model in relationships with patients, friends, and community members is important. The preceptorship is also your opportunity to incorporate teaching related to the ethical dilemmas that are a part of daily practice.

Student's Assessment

In the beginning of your precepting experience, it is important to determine the level of your student's knowledge. You should integrate into your teaching activities the student's knowledge and relevant past life experiences, which may include work, family, or volunteer experiences.

Teaching methods should vary to accommodate the student's individual learning style. Different students or circumstances will require that you modify your methods. Potential learning preferences include:

■ Socratic case presentations, which are often easily incorporated into a morning report or hospital rounds
■ small group discussions, which can be enriched by incorporating multiple disciplines
■ independent study, including textbooks, CD-ROMs, or the Internet
■ experiential or hands-on training
■ mini-lectures or brief didactic sessions

Creating a High-Quality Learning Experience

Once you have assessed your own teaching style, determined the student's preferred learning methods, and mutually agreed on your intended outcomes, you can work to create a quality learning experience (Whitman and

Optimal Learning

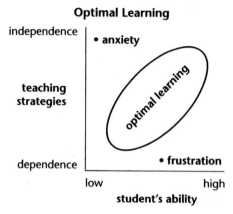

Figure 14.1. Matching teaching strategies and student abilities to create an optimal learning climate. A student on his or her first clerkship will benefit from dependent strategies to avoid anxiety, while a senior student will benefit from more independent strategies to avoid frustration.

Schwenk, 1995). The optimal learning climate matches a student's ability with the level of teacher involvement (Figure 14.1).

It is helpful to include direct observation of the student-patient interaction to best determine what knowledge, skills, or attitudes should be emphasized. Patients find this technique very acceptable and recognize this as physician contact time.

A variety of types of questions can be used to stimulate acquisition of knowledge. These include:

- *factual questions*, which can be helpful in quickly assessing the student's specific knowledge base (include both basic science and clinical questions)
- *broadening questions*, which attempt to enlarge the differential for a current problem and may involve a review of the general management of an acute problem

- *justifying questions*, which involve asking about specific treatment plans or medication side effects and will help you to determine the depth of the student's understanding
- *hypothetical questions*, which can help you use a single clinical encounter to assess other areas of student knowledge; this can be accomplished by rephrasing questions to change the age or gender of the patient or the specifics of the complaint
- *alternative questions*, which can be useful in helping students to recognize that there are many correct ways of treating patients; these questions also help in reviewing the natural history of the disease process

Various styles of teaching can be used to broaden your repertoire in different situations. As described by Quirk (1994) they are:

- *assertive*: the preceptor provides information
- *suggestive*: the alternatives are presented for the student
- *collaborative*: students are encouraged to do more problem solving
- *facilitative*: designed to promote more student self-understanding

By using the various types of questions and styles noted, you can adapt the way you teach to most effectively suit your student's needs as well as the intended teaching goal.

Once you have determined your student's abilities and learning style and have assessed your own teaching strategies, you are ready to apply your knowledge to individual teaching situations to provide an optimal environment for learning. Finally, by integrating the student's current abilities, your teaching style, and the desired goal, you are ready to apply yourself to teaching situations to provide an optimal environment for learning, as illustrated in Figure 14.1.

References

Irby, D. M. 1995. Teaching and learning in ambulatory care settings: A thematic review of the literature. *Academic Medicine* 70(10):898–931.

Quirk, M. E. 1994. *How to Learn and Teach in Medical School: A Learner-Centered Approach.* Springfield, Ill.: Charles C Thomas.

Swee, D. 1991. *Teaching Family Medicine in Medical School: A Companion to Education in Family Medicine.* The Society of Teachers of Family Medicine and the American Academy of Family Physicians, Kansas City, Mo.

Whitman, N., and Schwenk, T. L. 1995. *Preceptors as Teachers: A Guide to Clinical Teaching*, 2d ed. Department of Family and Preventive Medicine, University of Utah, School of Medicine, Salt Lake City, Utah.

■ 15

Formative Feedback

Katherine C. Krause, M.D.

Key Points

■ Providing feedback to your students is a critical part of improving your students' performance.

■ Feedback should be timely.

■ Feedback should be specific and behavior oriented.

Feedback is information based on direct observation of performance, which is reflected back to the learner without judgment about quality. Feedback offers repeated opportunities to modify behavior to improve clinical performance (Ende, 1983).

Learners need to know what they are doing well and to receive guidance on how they can improve. If students and residents are not provided with a mirror, they create their own images of how they are doing from incomplete or inaccurate clues. "You're doing fine" can be interpreted as "I am an honor student" rather than "You are performing at an appropriate level for your training." Learners complain that they do not get enough feedback from their preceptors, and the literature supports this concern. The two most frequent criticisms from students are lack of direction and lack of feedback. While learners should be encouraged to seek feedback, if they do not, we are still obliged to provide it. How can we do it effectively? By remembering the cardinal rules of feedback (Kaprielian and Gradeson, 1998).

■ Provide feedback as soon after an encounter as possible and make it behavior specific. It should concern what is said and done; how, not why a task is done. Attributing motives or making assumptions about why something occurred is not helpful in improving performance. Remember that behavior, by definition, can be changed; personality cannot. Give details about what was done well and what might have been done differently. Base feedback on factual information and observed performance. For example, you might observe: "When you pointed out to the patient that he had been able to quit smoking before, he seemed less discouraged about his ability to do so. What else could you do?"

- Ask the learners about which topics they would like feedback on, how they would like to receive it, and when (at the end of the day, with a chart review, or following an encounter).

- Focus your comments on the item that you view as most important for that patient encounter.

- Be brief and concise, but let the learner know specifics. For example, you might suggest to the student who goes into the exam room and takes an hour, "John, for the next patient I want you to gather as much history about the presenting problem as possible in ten minutes and then give me an oral summary. We will go in and do the physical exam together," or "This time I want to watch you do a more targeted history and physical within the patient's allotted time slot."

- Base feedback on a question the learner has formulated. Ask learners what they think they did well and what they did that could be improved. This approach often relieves you of the need to correct their behavior because they identify the problems and possible solutions. When students can do this self-evaluation, they can institute midcourse corrections, an important skill for the mature, self-directed learner.

- Provide feedback that is balanced and reinforces what they did well and that suggests improvements. Some preceptors use the one-minute manager technique: bad news followed by good news (or the reverse). Others use the Oreo, or sandwich, technique—good news wrapped around bad news—to make it more palatable. Use whichever is more comfortable for you, but be sure to provide feedback at regular intervals.
- Encourage two-way feedback. First you will need to reassure students that the learning environment is a risk-free climate in which it is safe to provide feedback toward improving your teaching skills. You could ask, "What am I doing that contributes to your learning? What should I consider doing differently to enhance your learning?"

When Should You Give Feedback?

Establish a learning contract with the student or resident at the beginning of the rotation, outlining mutual expectations for learning and performance. It is important to set up a midrotation meeting to discuss progress toward fulfilling the student's goals. Are both sides meeting their obligations? What more can the learner do to improve performance in the last half of the rotation? Should the contract be modified or expanded?

On a daily basis, informal feedback can occur when it is most convenient. Going over charts together at the end of a session serves as a reminder of specific points you want to convey to the learner. Note cards (3 × 5) with incidents jotted down or questions for the student to look up are helpful and can be pulled out at any time (e.g., between patients or over lunch). Example: "Today accomplished ellipse biopsy, edges well approximated, gave clear wound care instructions. Had read about melanomas. Needs to differentiate benign from malignant lesions."

Students can prepare talks on diagnosis and management of common ambulatory problems, and you can provide feedback in the car on the way to the hospital, or over coffee in the morning.

How Can You Take Time to Give Feedback and Still Manage to Maintain Productivity?

The University of Washington has developed an effective and popular five-step "microskills" model of clinical teaching (Neher et al., 1992) (see Chapter 29). It is learner centered and does not require the preceptor to be a fount of knowledge. It is designed to keep the encounter to less than five minutes and is highly efficient. This model reveals much about the facts learners use to make decisions and the decision-making process itself. The student is asked first to formulate a working diagnosis and then is probed for data or supporting evidence. The preceptor then states a general rule that applies to similar clinical situations. "Patients with cystitis usually have the following signs and symptoms." After the encounter, learners are asked to critique their performance. They may already be aware there was a problem. This interaction is an opportunity to acknowledge the problem and to seek out your recommendations on how to prevent repetitions in the future. If the student is unaware, the focus should still be on how to correct the problem rather than stating that the whole case was handled badly. The preceptor reinforces what the student did well in terms of specific behaviors: "You kept an open mind until the patient revealed her true agenda for the visit. You saved yourself and the patient time and unnecessary expense by getting to the heart of her concerns first." Mistakes are then corrected tactfully.

Scheduling your patients in waves helps build in time for feedback. Some preceptors schedule a 15-minute appointment with the learner midway through each half day for feedback and questions. Tell them your time is limited. "I can meet with you now for ten minutes. You can have five minutes to ask me questions, then I need five minutes to give you some feedback on the patient we saw together earlier this afternoon."

Learning to give effective feedback is a skill that, developed over time, is helpful not only in preparing competent physicians but also in negotiating with professional colleagues, raising your teenaged children, and strengthening partner relationships.

References

Ende, J. 1983. Feedback in clinical medical education. *Journal of the American Medical Association* 250:777–81.

Kaprielian, V., and Gradeson, M. 1998. Effective use of feedback. *Family Medicine* 30(6):406–7.

Neher, J., Gordon, K., Meyer, B., and Stevens, N. 1992. A five-step "microskills" model of clinical teaching. *Journal of the American Board of Family Practice* 5(4):419–24.

▪ 16

Summative Feedback, Evaluation, and Grading Students

L. Peter Schwiebert, M.D., and
William Bondurant, M.D.

Key Points

- ▪ Summative feedback guides students' acquisition of knowledge and skills.
- ▪ Well-delineated goals and objectives facilitate the evaluation of students.
- ▪ These are time-efficient methods of student evaluation.

In the broadest sense, feedback is the information a system uses to make adjustments in pursuit of a goal. In medical education, this occurs when a trainee receives insight into what he or she actually did vis-à-vis an intended result, thereby providing incentive for change. Feedback is information, is neutral, and is formative. Summative feedback is defined as the final assessment of a learning experience, the "final grade" on student strengths and weaknesses for the rotation. It usually is seen in the comments section of an evaluation form, and may or may not be discussed with the student. Summative feedback can be compared with formative feedback, which consists of frequent suggestions throughout the rotation on areas of accomplishment and areas needing improvement. In contrast, evaluation is judgmental (i.e., it addresses how well or poorly a learner performed, often in comparison with peers). Inasmuch as it provides a trainer's distillation of overall trainee performance, evaluation can also be called "summative feedback." The focus of this chapter is on both feedback and evaluation, with an emphasis on facilitating the development of effective clinicians.

Importance of Feedback

To appreciate the importance of summative feedback, it is helpful to consider what the training of students would be like in the absence of preceptor feedback. Certainly, a lack of feedback during clinical experiences decreases students' awareness both of what they are doing well and what needs improvement and therefore decreases the likelihood that students will act on those areas. In effect, lack of preceptor feedback leaves learners adrift and without reference points for their performance, thereby slowing the processes of clinical learning and skill acquisition. Ende (1983) describes potential repercussions of the absence of these external reference points of performance. To fill a feedback void, students begin attaching a significance to various internal and external cues that is often inappropriate. As they become more confident in evaluating their own performance (based on their own cues), they tend, as house officers, to downplay or disparage discordant external feedback (even if it is from supervisors) and resist any change except as dictated by their own cues.

With regular feedback, the learning environment is markedly different. If one views a clerkship as an apprenticeship, then feedback and evaluation provide an experienced clinician's (i.e., the "master's") perspective on what the apprentice is doing well and what needs work, thereby expediting development of the skills and behaviors modeled by the "master." Clinical feedback is global and addresses not only knowledge (which is evaluated on typical written examinations), but also such diverse areas as interpersonal skills and the ability to integrate and apply information in real-world clinical settings (Miller, 1990). As such, it is the most important feedback clinicians-in-training can receive. Finally, appropriate feedback conveys the preceptor's concern and interest, and because of the way it is delivered, such feedback facilitates openness to and eagerness for further feedback, rather than the denial found in a system where feedback is absent or poorly delivered.

Standards for Evaluating Students' Performance and Providing Feedback

On most clinical clerkships, the student's grade consists of several components, including performance on oral or written examinations, other assignments (case write-ups, case presentations, papers) and clinical performance. Although there are many approaches to evaluating student clinical performance, most address the following broad areas, which are worth keeping in mind when interacting with students:

- *attitude* (including participation, willingness to take responsibility or initiative, attendance, and dependability)
- *interpersonal skills* (including rapport with patients, peers, and staff)
- *knowledge base* (basic sciences, application of expected knowledge from prior clerkships, knowledge of practical assessment, and management of problems commonly encountered in family medicine)
- *history taking* (especially appropriate focused history for commonly encountered problems)
- *physical examination* (skill, accuracy, and appropriate focused exam for common problems)
- *assessment and management plan* (ability to interpret history, exam and lab studies, and to propose further

interventions, including patient education, testing, and follow-up)

■ *case presentation and write-up* (ability to organize and present information in a concise, cohesive narrative).

Many evaluation instruments provide a Likert scale (e.g., 1–9, where 9 = best, 1 = worst) in each of the above areas, coupled with descriptions of performance consistent with various levels on the scale. In addition, both in assigning a grade and planning experiences for students, it is important to take prior student experiences into account. It is helpful to know what prior clerkship or professional experiences a student has had and know the student's self-assessed skill levels for various cognitive or procedural aspects of the clerkship or preceptorship. Finally, patients are an invaluable and underutilized source of feedback on students' interpersonal skills, attitude, and professionalism; it is worth asking patients to share their feelings and perceptions both with students and with their preceptors.

Assessing student performance in the areas just mentioned is only part of a preceptor's job; at least as important is sharing these assessments with the student. Ende (1983) gave helpful guidelines for formulating and delivering feedback. These include providing feedback that is timely, based on firsthand data, limited in scope and addressing remediable behaviors, descriptive and not evaluative, and specific and dealing with decisions and actions rather than assumed intentions or interpretations. A helpful mnemonic for formulating and delivering feedback is TOLD AS (*t*imely, *o*bserved, *l*imited, *d*escriptive, *a*ctions, *s*pecific).

In addition, it is important to emphasize positive aspects of student performance in sharing feedback, and this can be done using the "sandwich" approach; that is, starting and ending with positives and fitting aspects needing improvement in between.

Providing Useful Feedback to Students in a Busy Office Practice

Even in a busy practice, evaluation of students' interpersonal skills and attitudes is usually not a big challenge, based on a review of nine years of evaluations by busy community preceptors participating in our decentralized third-year clerkship. Often, however, observations of interpersonal skills are limited to interactions with preceptors and staff, rather than with patients. Because of time constraints or a feeling that students already know how to interact appropriately with patients, students are not often observed interviewing and examining patients. Since this is the "doctor-patient relationship," it is a crucial determinant of students' success and patient satisfaction with them as clinicians. Put differently, brilliant students with poor interpersonal skills may find patients abandoning them for the physician down the block or across town. To assess interpersonal skills, preceptors should consider observing students as they interview and examine patients, provide students with feedback on these skills, and ask students to present in front of patients. This strategy gives students practice at so-called bedside presentation and allows preceptors to corroborate student findings.

Evaluating and providing students with feedback on data gathering and synthesis is a major challenge in a busy office practice and it is often not done well, owing to multiple competing tasks, the fast pace of office practice, and the absence of documentation of students' clinical decision-making. To improve this documentation (and lay the foundation for feedback), preceptors may find it helpful to jot notes to themselves about formative feedback shared with students at the end of a session or a day. A review of such notes from several sessions will indicate trends in strengths and weaknesses of the student's data gathering and decision-making and establish the basis for specific, helpful summative feedback. Alternatively, the preceptor may choose to use student write-ups as a feedback vehicle. The preceptor can ask students to jot down findings, assessment, and a plan as they interview patients, then hand these to the preceptor before presenting, so the preceptor can note areas of the history, physical, assessment, and plan included or omitted by the student. These student and preceptor notes serve as a template for both end-of-session feedback on student decision-making and the dictated or written progress note.

Other tools with well-documented utility in providing feedback on student clinical skills include video- or audiotaped patient interviews conducted by students (Kihm et al., 1991). These tapes facilitate review and feedback of specific or critical incidents in decision-making that may otherwise be missed in a busy office practice. Clinical simulations (e.g., standardized patients, objective structured clinical examinations) and the oral examination also facilitate the feedback process (Schwiebert and Davis, 1993). The latter are case-based ways of evaluating affective skills, communication, patient education, and clinical reasoning in a more structured, less harried environment than the typical office setting.

In summary, feedback and evaluation are essential to the development of the effective, capable, and honest clinicians all of us hope to see inheriting the mantle of the medical profession. In formulating feedback, it is helpful to internalize a set of criteria, keeping the criteria and a few basic guidelines for delivering feedback in mind when you share this information with students. Finally, it is possible to do all these things effectively in a busy office practice.

References

Ende, J. 1983. Feedback in clinical medical education. *Journal of the American Medical Association* 250:777–81.

Kihm, J. T., Brown, J. T., Divine, G. W., and Linzer, M. 1991. Quantitative analysis of the outpatient oral case presentation: piloting a method. *Journal of General Internal Medicine* 6:233–36.

Miller, G. E. 1990. The assessment of clinical skills/competence/performance. *Academic Medicine* 65 (Suppl.):S63–67.

Schwiebert, L. P., and Davis, A. B. 1993. Increasing inter-rater agreement on a family medicine clerkship oral examination: a pilot study. *Family Medicine* 25:182–85.

Advising from a Preceptor's Perspective

Laeth Nasir, M.D.

Key Points
- The advisee-advisor relationship is highly valued by students.
- Students will seek advice about career choices and personal matters.
- Effective advice is tailored to the learning stage and background of the student.

A major part of becoming a physician involves absorbing the advice of teachers. We all treasure memories of timely and valuable guidance given by wise mentors. Many have less fond memories of advice given thoughtlessly or carelessly by others. Having benefited from good advice in our careers, it is natural for us to want to provide the same to the students we teach. Giving useful advice requires that you recall your own feelings and concerns as a medical student, while recognizing that in some ways the pressures students face today are unique.

Many students consider a number of possible careers in medical school. Ideally, a field is chosen to match personal talents and interests to the demands of the specialty. In reality, this process is often modified through expectations of family and friends, opportunity, and circumstance. The counsel of an experienced advisor is invaluable in helping a student decide which career might be most congruent with their own needs and strengths. Medical students are not exempt from issues such as relationships, lifestyle, and finances, and might profit from a mentor's advice. Preceptors will often find themselves sup-plying advice on personal matters if a good relationship with the student is achieved.

The most potent but least recognized forms of advice are the attitudes and behaviors displayed by the preceptor toward others. Medical students are disproportionately influenced by this kind of "advice," since they are in the process of assimilating attitudes as well as knowledge. Physicians who are disparaging toward patients or subor-dinates, and who display racism, sexism, or other dis-agreeable traits are transmitting powerful messages. Atti-tudes that are sufficiently discordant with the student's past opinions and experiences are usually rejected, to-gether with any useful information or experiences that the preceptor may have been able to offer. Conversely, physicians who model traits such as honesty and equa-nimity are often rewarded by seeing their students un-consciously begin to display these behaviors in their own interactions with patients.

Exposure to clinical medicine leads many students to reexamine their relationship to medicine, no matter how well prepared they may be for the experience. Most stu-dents revel in the fresh challenges provided by the clini-cal setting. Others may feel intimidated or disillusioned by their interactions with patients. The most common reaction students have is expressed in the sentence, "I always thought I wanted to be a . . . , now I'm not so sure." The preceptor may be sought out as a resource to help clarify the student's feelings about the new environ-ment, and help the student to identify what challenges they may encounter in future clinical work.

It is important to consciously set aside some time, ideally after each clinical encounter, but more realistically in a busy office, at the end of the day, to "debrief" the student. Initially, specific questions regarding the encounter are answered. If it seems appropriate, some general questions might be posed. How did the student feel about the encounter? What feelings were engendered by certain patients? Did any case have particular resonance? Did the student have a particular aptitude for or enjoyment of certain aspects of the encounter? This kind of open-ended probe is a useful way to use the clinical encounter both as a tool for teaching medical science and as a catalyst to encourage the student to consider the more subjective aspects of the art of medicine. "Breaking the ice" in this way signals to the student that you are open to discussing important issues.

When asked for advice, keeping some general guidelines in mind will help. First, and most important, what question is being asked? Careful consideration of the content as well as the context of the question is important. Is the student asking for feedback? Is the advisee covertly asking for permission to do something, such as to consider a career change? Or is reflective listening the best service that can be provided? The latter option is a useful default that always has some value.

The next point to remember is that good advice should primarily meet the needs of the advisee. Some advisors may use their status to vent or engage in some other self-centered activity. Obviously, this serves the advisee poorly. In addition, attempts at self-aggrandizement are usually transparent to the student.

The final important element of giving good advice is to tailor it to the advisee's background and stage in training. Specific advice given to a premedical or beginning student is different from that given to a senior student or resident. Giving personalized advice is similar to orienting a naive traveler in a foreign land. Specific queries must be answered and individual needs anticipated. Does the country have unfamiliar customs that need to be learned? Are there subtle features in the terrain that, once recognized, offer the voyager unique opportunities to learn and discover? Are there unfamiliar dangers that should be emphasized? It is particularly important to adapt information to fit the individual student's background. Your own knowledge of the individual and their stage of training or development is the best guide.

Having considered the above factors, it is important to speak your mind when advice is requested. If the question is of a specific nature, for example, the process of applying to a certain residency program, the answer is usually straightforward. If the question is more ambiguous, such as deciding on a medical specialty, it is important to clarify that there is no "right" answer. You can refer your student to a number of excellent books about selecting a specialty (Taylor, 1992; Iserson, 1996). Your own strong biases (if you have any) should be presented, so long as you make it clear that there may be other points of view that the advisee may want to consider. It is nearly impossible to give what would be considered purely "neutral" advice on any topic, and it is one of the inescapable hazards of giving or receiving advice.

Second only to the bond between physician and patient, the student-teacher bond is one of the most durable in medicine. In large part, precepting medical students is an endeavor that consists of the transfer of implicit and explicit advice from teacher to student. Planning for the latter, and self-reflection for the former will make the process rewarding and productive for both parties.

References

Iserson, K.V. 1996. *Getting into a Residency*, 4th ed. Tucson, Ariz.: Galen Press.

Taylor, A. 1992. *How to Choose a Medical Specialty,* 3d ed. Philadelphia: W. B. Saunders.

▪ 18

Dealing with Learners at Different Levels

A. Patrick Jonas, M.D., and
Laurence C. Bauer, M.S.W., M.Ed.

Key Points
- Students progress through predictable stages of learner development.
- Knowledge of the characteristics of these stages will improve your teaching.

Studies examining how we learn indicate that learners progress through stages of development (Scandura, 1974). The first stage is the *neophyte* stage. The learning of neophytes is slow and incremental. They must focus their attention in a step-by-step fashion, which is similar to using a procedural manual. Neophytes need basic knowledge and skills and exposure to simple cases and situations so they can discern the rules of operation (how the steps work as a whole). Because neophytes do not see the overall patterns (big picture), they need someone more experienced to frame the problems and issues that require attention. This is a mechanical stage where performance is slow and tedious.

The *apprentice*, on the other hand, has learned the fundamental skills and needs practice with increasingly more difficult cases. Rather than repetitious practice with the basics, apprentices learn from the feedback received on their routines. Apprentices also need a standard against which to compare their performance. As apprentices gain confidence, concern with efficiency increases. An apprentice is a consistent performer within a given area, but bogs down with unusual or complex cases or situations.

At the *master* stage, performance is integrated, smooth, graceful, and almost automatic. The master recognizes patterns and has a set of rules to self-critique their performance. At this level, performers can extrapolate from their own experience to approach new and unusual problems. Concern with efficiency and effectiveness is balanced. The master seeks exposure to variation to stimulate learning. The opportunity to teach is rewarding because it supports the master's continued learning.

Experienced physicians have learned to reduce the mental strain of performing a complex set of behaviors by creating routines and habits that synthesize problem-solving and interpersonal behaviors, such as those involved in an office visit, into a routine or a style that allows the physician to effectively care for substantial numbers of individuals and families each day. The challenge for experienced physicians is to learn how to break down their mastery into digestible units and teaching strategies that can facilitate and not overwhelm the neophyte and apprentice-level learners.

We have used a competency-based education approach in which the key competencies needed to perform the office visit are articulated (Bell, Kozakowski, and Winter 1997; Carkhuff, 1978). The competencies are broken down into steps and skills that match a learner's level of development. Practice opportunities also fit the learner's level of ability. Feedback is directed to the learner's use of skill drills, and the degree of difficulty of the learning is increased as the learner progresses.

A skill drill is an activity involving a discrete set of behaviors that focuses the learner's attention on a specific area of performance. For example, learners who need to improve their ability to elicit a history of present illness are directed to focus their attention during the history taking by seeking CODIERS information from the patient (*c*ourse, *o*nset, *d*uration, *i*ntensity, *e*xacerbations, *r*emissions, associated symptoms). This mnemonic provides a focal point for practicing a task that most neophytes can learn fairly quickly, thus supporting the learner's experience of success. After the student is comfortable with this task, additional skill drills are introduced so the learner gradually expands his or her repertoire of data-gathering and decision-making skills. The SPIT model, described below, is another example of a skill drill.

One approach to personalizing your response as a preceptor for different levels of learners is to determine the developmental level of the student. First-year students should be able to clarify the patient's chief complaint; elicit a history of present illness (HOPI); and obtain a past, family, and social history. The second-year student will have a neophyte level of competence in a few areas of pathophysiology, in addition to first-year skills. They should be able to ask many patients some questions reflective of a diagnostic consideration (hypothesis-driven interview). Third-year students should have second-year skills and the ability to generate a differential diagnosis. They should be able to use their skills to do a hypothesis-driven clinical encounter with about half of the patients seen early in their academic year and 75 percent of the patients later in the year as they become more experienced. They should write a "SOAP" note, and the preceptor may need to help with this to best support the differential diagnosis and assessment. Their plan might be very weak. The students may need lots of help to understand the pertinent positive and negative information that should be included in the note. Learners should be able to present the information to you in a time-efficient manner with guidance.

Fourth-year students should demonstrate all these skills; they may occasionally have some difficulty with more complex patients. They should be expected to write a SOAP note and to present the patient in an efficient manner. Their plan should be "good" to "very good" for about one-third to one-half of the patients they see. Each student will have personal variations and each medical school will have variations in the knowledge and skills expected. You should meet with the student at the beginning of the clerkship to clarify his or her knowledge and skill level. Plan to meet weekly to review the student's progress.

Medical students differ in many respects, especially in their clinical knowledge, skills, and attitudes. Being sensitive to core clinical skills of the student, such as making a differential diagnosis, adds to the preceptor's ability to effectively respond to learners of different levels while teaching several key principles. We like to teach the third- and fourth-year learners to have a four-part differential diagnosis using the mnemonic SPIT (*s*erious; *p*robably; *i*nteresting; *t*reatable assessments, disorders, conditions, or diseases). Before entering the exam room, we ask them to review the information available (on the daily schedule and in the medical record of the patient, including problem list, medication list, demographic information, vital signs, chief complaint for today, and the last visit entry) and "SPIT" out a differential diagnosis. For example, a patient who is a 19-year-old male college sophomore comes to your office with the chief complaint of painful throat, swollen neck, and fatigue for two weeks. His last visit was for a precollege physical 16 months ago. The student might put the following on a Post-it note: S–leukemia, P–mononucleosis, I–aplastic anemia, T–strep throat.

We ask the students to paste their "SPIT" in the chart on a Post-it note at least once a day so we can provide feedback about it. Many learners are hesitant to do this because they think there is a "right" answer. Others enjoy the exercise, especially hearing your SPIT and comparing it with theirs. Initially, the student will include a lot of items reflective of their last clinical rotation. Toward the end of the rotation, they should be able to think of broader assessments, consistent with community practice (e.g., S–alcoholism, P–malnutrition, I–leukemia, and T–poverty for a 90-year-old male, widower, edentulous patient with the chief complaint of swollen glands who lives alone in a mobile home). This patient's problem list includes alcoholism, hypertension, and hypoalbuminemia. Included in the last medical record note was "electricity will be turned off unless we document his medical needs for having electricity."

During the second week of the rotation, we have the students discuss how their SPIT changes during the clinical encounter as they interact with and examine the patient. We also discuss how our SPIT differs from theirs, noting that the "probably" and "treatable" parts of the differential quickly become the focus of the preceptor, while the student is very knowledgeable about the "serious" and "interesting" elements. Many students underestimate the potential for serious illness resulting from common complaints in community practice, while others are convinced that every headache is a brain tumor. They need to hear about your experience and knowledge to understand community practice at a novice level.

During the third week, we ask the students to integrate the patient's theory about the etiology for the chief complaint into their differential diagnosis, learning how to "SPIT with the patient." The patient's theory must be included in the student's presentation. This process reaffirms the importance of the doctor-patient relationship in community practice, especially as it pertains to making an accurate assessment and having it align with the belief system of the patient, while respecting the patient's self-knowledge.

The fourth and subsequent weeks are used to expand their SPIT by at least once a day writing a SPIT before, during, and after seeing the patient. This process helps assess how the students' thinking changes as they gain more information. We may add family issues into the more advanced SPIT (based on the patient's family life cycle, genetic conditions, the biopsychosocial model, and the "family SPIT"). Other principles can fit into variations of SPIT as the student demonstrates advancement through the rotation.

Throughout a community rotation, using the community practice differential diagnosis with a model such as SPIT can allow the preceptor to be in touch with the developmental level of each student. The preceptor's personalized responses to student differential diagnoses can enable students to advance in knowledge, skills, and attitudes in a stepwise fashion. The preceptor can rapidly identify student strengths and needs relative to the principles and content of our specialty. They may advance from novice first-year students to become apprentices by their fourth-year elective clerkship, by learning from you, the expert clinician.

References

Bell, H., Kozakowski, S., and Winter, R. 1997. Competency-based education in family practice. *Family Medicine* 29(10):701–4.

Carkhuff, R. 1978. *The Skills of Teaching*. Amherst, Mass.: Human Resource Development Press.

Scandura, J. 1974. Mathematical problem solving. *American Mathematical Monthly* 81(3):273–80.

▪ 19

Dealing with the Problem Learner

Norman B. Kahn Jr., M.D.

Key Points

Problems between teachers and learners most often fall into one of the following categories:

- The teacher may be an excellent and successful practitioner but have limited pedagogical skills and teaching experience (category 1).
- The learner may be unskilled and inexperienced in showing empathy, developing rapport, and relating to people as patients (category 2).
- The learner may be underprepared for what is being taught (category 3).
- The learner may learn comparatively slowly (category 4).
- The learner may have adequate knowledge but be technically relatively unskilled (category 5).
- The learner may be insecure, as manifested by behaviors as disparate as hostility, overconfidence, disorganization, dependence, or overwork (category 6).
- Less commonly, the learner may be impaired by mental illness or substance abuse (category 7).

Identification

Problems between teacher and learner may be identified by direct observation of the teacher, particularly when the difficulties are in relating to patients or the act of learning (categories 2 through 5). Problematic behavior (category 6) may first be identified by office staff. As in establishing a treatment plan for a patient, effective interventions are dependent on making an accurate diagnosis of the learning problem:

- Is the preceptor struggling to teach what he knows how to do well in practice (category 1)?
- Is the learner not communicating an understanding of the patient's point of view?
- Is the physician receiving complaints from patients about the learner (category 2)?
- Is the learner in "over his head," or expected to perform in a manner that exceeds his or her experience or level of training (category 3)?
- Is the learner making progress but much more slowly than the teacher expected or than has been the teacher's experience with the learner's peers (category 4)?
- Is the learner perceived by the teacher as bright, with an adequate fund of knowledge, but struggling with office procedures, charting, or other aspects of care (category 5)?
- Is the learner frustrating for the office staff or the teacher because of the learner's attitude or behavior, seeming lack of organization, dependence on the teacher to make decisions, or because of working long hours without commensurate productivity (category 6)?
- Does the learner display deterioration in personal appearance, withdrawal, unexplained absences, decreasing quality of or interest in work, marked behavioral changes, risk-taking behavior, tearfulness, agitation, mood swings, or other "signal behaviors" suggestive of substance abuse or mental illness (category 7)?

Intervention

Inexperienced Teacher

Category 1: If the problem is primarily in the skills and experience of the teacher, this book, workshops at regional and national meetings, and other faculty development experiences should be recommended.

Most of the problems between teachers and learners fall into categories 2 through 6, namely, clinical competence, or attitude and behavior problems. Intervening with each of these problems begins with objective, nonjudgmental confrontation and feedback (see chapters 15 and 16).

Clinical Competence Problems

Category 2: If the problem is in establishing a therapeutic doctor-patient relationship, including empathy, rapport, and communication skills, modeling is an effective intervention. After preparing the student for what he or she should observe, the teacher should demonstrate empathy, establishing rapport, and creating a meaningful doctor-patient relationship. Following this activity, the teacher should observe the learner and comment constructively on the learner's implementation of these same behaviors.

Categories 3 and 4: If the problem is an underprepared or slowly progressing learner, the teacher may need to take a step back to reestablish reasonable expectations. If progress is steady but slow, it will be important to communicate both to the learner and to his or her supervisors that the learner is progressing, but you should also establish expectations that are reasonable. If a learning disability is suspected, appropriate testing should be considered.

Category 5: A learner who has adequate knowledge but is technically unskilled may need to focus on technical aspects of the practice of medicine, such as procedures or charting. Some students are less technically adept, particularly with procedures, and may ultimately choose to focus their practices on the more cognitive aspects of medicine.

Learners with problems in categories 2 through 5 may be easier for the teacher to confront in that these skills are central to the role of the physician. In contrast, learners with attitude or behavioral problems in category 6 may be more frustrating for the teacher. Learners with problems in category 2 may engender patient complaints, whereas learners with problems in category 6 will likely engender complaints from staff.

Attitude and Behavior Problems

Category 6: The key to addressing problems of attitude and behavior in the learner may lie in an assumption on the part of the teacher that whether the learner is aware of it or not, he or she may be insecure in the role of physician. This insecurity may be manifested as "acting out," hostility, or complaining, whereas some learners will overcompensate and exhibit overconfidence. Some students are simply unable to be adequately organized or to make an independent decision. Still others seem to take forever, working long hours while making little progress.

Objective, nonjudgmental confrontation and feedback is the first step with learners who manifest attitude or behavior problems. Such feedback should focus on specific observed behaviors, including their acceptability and their natural consequences (not threats). The teacher may want to empathize with the learner, reflecting on how the teacher has behaved when feeling overwhelmed.

People have a tendency to do more of what they are told they do well. Therefore, after confrontation and identification, it is often useful for the teacher to reinforce the strengths and successes of the learner while teaching new skills one at a time, with positive reinforcement. The problem of dealing with impaired physicians and learners (category 7) is beyond the scope of this chapter.

When It Doesn't Work

If the learner's progress does not meet the teacher's expectations or if the learner's behavior continually frustrates the teacher, the teacher is encouraged to first revisit the descriptive categories of problems between teachers and learners. Can the teacher change or improve the focus or method of instruction (category 1)? Is the learner a knowledgeable clinician but simply relatively unskilled in relating to people (category 2), or is the learner an inadequate clinician for his or her level of training (categories 3 and 4)? Is the learner knowledgeable enough, and even able to relate well to patients, but difficult when interacting with the teacher or staff (category 6)?

The teacher is encouraged to seek guidance and assistance from the learner's supervisors at the medical school. In this way, the problems can be called to the attention of department or residency staff and further attempts can be made to assist the learner in achieving the goals of the educational experience.

The relationship between a single learner and preceptor in the office is among the best of the learning situations in medical education. Many focused interventions, including required supervision, one-on-one precepting, and reviewing individual encounters, occur naturally in the preceptor-learner office environment. A preceptor can significantly enhance the experience by identifying one or more patients who are willing to assume an adjunct teacher role with the learner. With a little focused prompting, many patients will welcome the opportunity to serve as teachers. If the teacher asks the patient to help the student learn the physical exam for the patient's condition (e.g., arthritis), the patient functions similarly to a "standardized patient" in a more formal learning environment. Similarly, patients may be prompted to give feedback to the learner regarding those behaviors that demonstrate empathy or establish rapport.

Students overwhelmingly appreciate the experience of working one-on-one with a preceptor in a community-based practice. This setting is, after all, the "real" practice of medicine, which is each student's goal. The experience can be substantially enhanced through supportive feedback, including praise for skills and behaviors that contribute to learning or effective practice.

It may be easier for the teacher early in training if the learning objectives are focused on the teacher as role model. Later in training, when learning objectives include the acquisition of basic clinical skills, the teacher shifts from being a role model to serving as a skill facilitator. When the relationship between the teacher and learner is less than smooth, the teacher has a unique opportunity to adequately identify the nature of the problem and begin potentially effective interventions. A successful intervention with a learner who is having problems can be one of the most rewarding experiences for the teacher and a critical experience for the learner.

■ IV

Organization of the
Preceptorship Curriculum

■ 20

The Ideal Preceptorship

Jeffrey A. Stearns, M.D.

Key Points

Elements of the ideal preceptorship include:
- a positive, educationally oriented work environment
- appropriate teaching facilities
- a clear setting of goals and expectations
- regular feedback and timely evaluation

As medical education moves to the ambulatory environment, there will be increased use of community sites for preceptorships. The answer to the question "What is the ideal preceptorship?" is likely to be "It depends on . . . ." In an effort to avoid this quandary, this chapter focuses on those characteristics that lead to superior experiences for all participants and that generate the best outcomes. Many of these elements will be addressed in greater detail in subsequent chapters.

Bowen et al. (1997) describe a methodology for addressing quality issues in ambulatory education. These issues include:
- the educational environment of the preceptorship (positive, supportive attitudes of staff; opportunities to work with the care team)
- physical aspects (exam rooms, teaching space)
- characteristics of teachers (clinical competence, teaching skills, teacher-learner ratio)
- characteristics of learners (level of training, approach to experience)

- learning resources (appropriate numbers of patients, case mix, instructional aids, established curriculum)
- service (balance of patient care and learning opportunities)

In an extensive review of the literature on teaching and learning in ambulatory care settings, Irby (1995) called for increased continuity of the learner-teacher-patient triad; more opportunities for collaborative and self-directed learning; and strengthening of assessment and feedback and faculty development. He suggested that teaching will improve if faculty (preceptors) implement the following practices:

- Set clear and realistic expectations.
- Model and teach to the learner's needs.
- Observe the learner's performance and give specific feedback.
- Encourage independent learning and reflection.
- Supplement clinical instruction with readings, conferences, and monitoring.
- Create a positive learning environment.
- Reflect on and improve teaching.

Ullian, Bland, and Simpson (1994) identified characteristics of effective clinical teachers-preceptors. They serve as positive role models, demonstrating knowledge, clinical competence, and good rapport with patients. They are effective supervisors, providing learning opportunities and constructive feedback for students. Excellent teachers are enthusiastic and interested in their teaching role. They are accessible and take an active part in the learning process. Finally, they are supportive people—easy to work with, friendly, helpful, and caring. With this overview, it is possible to set forth some key elements of a quality preceptorship.

Setting Goals

It is key at the outset to establish goals. This element has three components: the goals of the preceptorship, the preceptor's goals, and the learner's goals. It is critical that the preceptorship have a defined curriculum with clear goals and objectives that are appropriate for the setting, the preceptor, and the student. In addition, it is important that the preceptor articulate specific expectations for the experience. Finally, the learners must clarify their own expectations for the preceptorship. These three elements must be considered before the preceptorship starts, allowing a specific and explicit learning contract to be developed. This contract should be periodically revisited and adjusted over the course of the preceptorship, allowing for growth and flexibility.

Environment

Implicit in Bowen's quality indicators are elements of the learning environment. There must be adequate space for the learners. Resources that promote high-quality learning include adequate patient numbers and a case mix appropriate for the level of the learner. Access to current textbooks, journals, instructional materials, and online resources is important. Given that a supportive environment is critical to quality learning, it is key that the entire team involved in the preceptorship understand the goals and facilitate the experience. This team includes all of the office personnel and other stakeholders (i.e., clinicians and employers) in the delivery of the care. Positive "buy-in" and collaboration means that all participants understand and work together to balance the service and learning aspects of the preceptorship.

Orientation

Another critical element of a high-quality preceptorship experience is the student orientation. Many students are unfamiliar with the office setting because most of their previous experience has been hospital based. The fast pace of patient care in the office is often bewildering. It is important to present the learner with a road map: who the personnel are, what they do, where things are in the office (exam room organization), how the schedule operates, and the demographics of the patient population. It is important to orient the student to the organization of charts and to give them key information about their scheduled patients. The comfort level of the student is associated with the quality of learning. The involvement of the student is dependent on their level of learning, but should be progressive over the course of the preceptorship.

Observation and Feedback

Although much can be inferred from the student's presentation, it is important to directly observe the student to provide performance-based feedback. This observation does not mean watching the entire H&P, but rather taking the opportunity to observe the student at critical points in the process. This can be done by agreeing on a strategy for observation before the encounter. Students learn best by focused, specific, and timely commentary on their performance.

Evaluation

Evaluation is the final component in ensuring a high-quality experience. If the goals of all the participants have been set at the beginning of the preceptorship, and revisited and adjusted periodically during the experience, evaluation can be rather straightforward. If the goals have been explicit and feedback has been specific and timely, there should be no surprises. Understanding, agreement, and communication before and during the preceptorship make for a high-caliber evaluation.

For some time, many of us have recognized that community preceptorships can add significant value to medical education. Fortunately, this is now being acknowledged by academic institutions. As in all aspects of our professional lives, quality is being demanded. Attention paid up-front to the elements of a quality preceptorship—goal setting, environment, orientation, observation, and feedback and evaluation—will ensure that an ideal preceptorship is provided.

References

Bowen, J., Stearns, J., Dohner, C., Blackman, J., and Simpson, D. 1997. Defining and evaluating quality for ambulatory care educational programs. *Academic Medicine* 72:506–10.

Irby, D. 1995. Teaching and learning in ambulatory care settings: a thematic review of the literature. *Academic Medicine* 70:898–931.

Ullian, J., Bland, C., and Simpson, D. 1994. An alternative approach to defining the role for the clinical teacher. *Academic Medicine* 69:832–38.

Reinventing the Community-Based Preceptorship

Cynthia A. Irvine, M.Ed., and William B. Shore, M.D.

Key Point
- The community preceptorship has moved beyond the teaching of the physical examination and medical history and includes competencies focused in the office, hospital, home, and community.

There is little doubt that precepting in an office-based setting has become more challenging. Academic medical centers are making more requests for community-based teaching at the same time that managed care is demanding that preceptors see more patients. For many physicians, precepting a student may result in seeing fewer patients or working a longer day. Even with these pressures, community preceptors continue to value teaching medical students, but if they are to continue precepting, they must develop creative approaches to teaching. The scope of what has been traditionally defined as an office-based preceptorship must be broadened.

In the past, the traditional office-based preceptorship was largely focused on physical examination and history-taking skills, and the educational relationship usually involved just two participants, the preceptor and the student. Contemporary practice demands that students learn far more than where to put the stethoscope. A reinvented preceptorship curriculum consists of what we call "multiple menus and venues": more options for what is taught, who does the actual teaching, and how and where teaching takes place. The result is greater flexibility for the busy preceptor, and greater exposure to the context of clinical practice for the student.

The scope of the reinvented preceptorship curriculum might be viewed as concentric circles, each representing a "venue," or arena for teaching (Figure 21.1). In each teaching arena, a variety of knowledge, attitudes, and skills (K-A-S) can be taught by a variety of members of the health care team. The following are examples.

Direct Patient Care

Participants:
Student with preceptor and other medical staff nurses, physician's assistants, technicians, social workers, and others

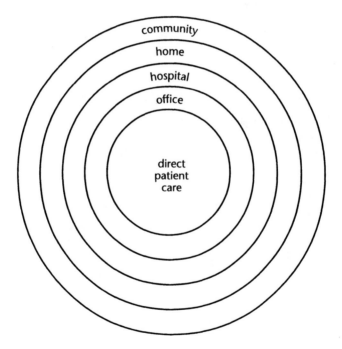

Figure 21.1. Scope of the preceptorship.

Knowledge:
- understanding of primary care and continuity of care
- understanding of what each professional discipline offers

Attitudes:
- respectful approach to all patients, cultures, groups, and medical disciplines
- appreciation for balance of communication and relational skills with technical expertise
- appreciation of primary care as challenging but "doable" and rewarding

Skills:
- basic physical exam and communication skills
- working as colleagues with different disciplines

Office

Participants:
Student with practice manager, receptionist or office assistant, and others

Knowledge:
- how office functions; who does what
- medical record procedures
- access to care, insurance issues, and managed care

Attitudes:
- respectful communication with all members of health care team
- appreciation for importance of practice management

Skills:
- responsive communication with nonmedical team members
- negotiation; how to create change effectively and appropriately

Hospital

Participants:
Student with preceptor, nurses, social workers, hospital administrators, patients, and families
Knowledge:
- role of hospital in continuity of care
- how preceptor incorporates hospital care into schedule
- relationship between generalist, specialist, and hospitalist
- understanding the course of serious illness
- insurance coverage for hospitalization

Attitudes:
- perspective on inpatient and outpatient medicine
- impact of hospitalization on patient and family
- impact of insurance issues on quality of care and length of stay

Skills:
- physical exam and history-taking skills

Home

Participants:
Student with home care nurse and other team members
Knowledge:
- impact of aging or chronic illness on patient and family
- impact of home environment on health and safety
- understanding of family systems
- contributions of other disciplines such as home health nursing and physical and occupational therapy
- teamwork

Attitudes:
- appreciation for the special contribution of the home visit to the doctor-patient relationship and the doctor's understanding of a patient's situation

Skills:
- history taking
- use of basic screening and health promotion tools
- functional and home assessment
- communication and interaction with team members, patients, and family

Community

(Defined as the preceptor's practice in the context of the larger community)

Participants:
Student with community leaders, agencies, and patients

Knowledge:
- impact of culture, socioeconomic status, and location on health care, access to care, and public health issues
- community resources and opportunities for intervention
- principles of community-oriented primary care (COPC)

Attitudes:
- acceptance of different perspectives on medical care (e.g., alternative healers)
- appreciation of strengths in community
- importance of other community resources
- acceptance that we (medical providers) may be outsiders and have much to learn from the community

Skills:
- how to identify and work with resources outside of the medical office

- how to motivate patients to use resources and how to educate ourselves about those resources (Fadiman, 1997)

A more broadly defined primary care preceptorship is clearly in step with contemporary practice. Sharing teaching responsibilities with others can also significantly minimize the perceived "burden" of precepting and create an enhanced learning experience for the student. Redefining the objectives and the means by which to accomplish them will result in improved teaching and learning and better prepared, more humane physicians.

It is critical, however, that *one* preceptor coordinate the various "menus and venues" and provide cohesion for the student's experience. The way in which a preceptor conveys satisfaction (or dissatisfaction) with contemporary medical practice can have a dramatic impact on the impressionable medical student. Preceptors must be aware of the effect that subtle comments or nonverbal communication of discontent can have on a student. The demonstration of a positive attitude toward patients and the practice of medicine can be the most significant influence on a student's career choice (Ambrozy et al., 1997).

References

Ambrozy, D., Irby, D., Bowen, J., Burack, J., Carline, J., and Stritter, F. 1997. Role models' perceptions of themselves and their influence on students' speciality choices. *Academic Medicine* 72:1119–21.

Fadiman, A. 1997. *The Spirit Catches You and You Fall Down: A Hmong Child, Her American Doctors and the Collision of Two Cultures*. New York: Farrar, Straus and Giroux.

■ 22

Costs of Precepting and How to Decrease Them

Lili Church, M.D., Gregory A. Doyle, M.D., and Thomas Greer, M.D., M.P.H.

Key Points

- Most studies suggest that precepting a medical student adds, on average, an hour to the workday.
- Although precepting may take additional time, the use of appropriate orientation, scheduling, and supervision can minimize any adverse financial impact.
- Preceptors gain significant nonmonetary rewards from their teaching efforts.

Precepting medical students has costs as well as many benefits for the physician. The benefits can be in the areas of reputation, intellectual stimulation, new learning, and personal satisfaction. The costs are in terms of time and money.

Time

Most studies suggest that physicians who precept a medical student add about 60 minutes to their workday. Preceptor time is required to orient the student to the clinic, including introductions to staff, patients, and colleagues. Teaching tasks include listening to student presentations, waiting for the student to finish with a patient, seeing patients or doing procedures with students, and giving mini-lectures or testing a student's knowledge. Many preceptors postpone their administrative duties to the end of their day. Time may be taken up in reviewing student chart dictations and coordinating follow-up phone calls, test results, or labs. At some sites, an extra effort is made to include students in professional or social events. A formal evaluation of students requires additional time, as do the informal tasks of advising and monitoring. In the minority of cases, when a significant student problem is identified, time for consultation with the student's medical school is needed to explore and develop strategies to address the area of concern. The clinic staff expends time in helping students with orientation and responding to their questions or need for assistance. Efficiency in moving patients through rooms may also be impeded.

Money

Although precepting students definitely requires extra time, it does not necessarily entail a loss of revenue. Some studies show that practices generate one to two fewer patient visits per day, whereas other studies conclude there is no loss in the number of patients seen or in gross charges. Indeed, experienced students can actually make it possible for a practice site to see more, not fewer, patients.

When precepting hours are translated into monetary compensation, the financial costs of teaching become visible. Paying $60 to $75 per hour for the 1.0–1.2 extra hours per day required to precept translates into costs between $1,254 and $1,754 for a four-week rotation (Ricer, Van Horne and Filak, 1997; Ricer, Filak, and David, 1998). This cost includes teaching time only and not preparation time, potential revenue lost because of fewer patients, extra staffing, or other expenses.

Cost Variables

Variable factors that influence the costs of precepting include the practice, the site, the student, and the preceptor. The costs of precepting will be influenced by the experience of the student and the style of the preceptor.

Students' individual interests, experience, and talents are diverse. Students in their fourth year or late in their third year will have more skills than students early in their third year. Similarly, students with previous health care expertise, for example, former nurses or paramedics, usually make the transition to ambulatory medicine quickly and contribute sooner to the monetary gain of a practice. The longer a rotation, the greater the opportunity for a practice site to benefit from a student. As with every rotation, the initial weeks are a time of transition and present a steep learning curve. Extending the length of a rotation may allow the early loss of productivity to be balanced by later gains.

A preceptor's experience, style, and interests will also affect costs. For instance, some educators have observed that the more frequently a physician precepted students, the less significant the effect of students on the physician's efficiency. These gains may be attributed to physicians learning to structure their time better to accommodate patient care and teaching. Patients become more comfortable with the presence of students and this decreases the time required for introductions and explanations.

A preceptor's style with patients is sometimes mirrored in his or her style with students. For example, a good listener usually listens well to patients and students alike. An efficient provider commonly covers much ground in a short time with students as well as with patients. The physician who teaches by example relies on modeling more than verbal explanation with both patients and students.

These styles translate into time and money. Recognition of his or her own natural style enables a physician preceptor to adjust this style to fit different circumstances. Different styles are associated with different goals. A savvy preceptor can carefully choose how to invest teaching time, electing on one occasion to closely supervise a student doing a new activity while on another allowing the student more independence. A preceptor may invest extra time in mentoring a particular student but at other times give this goal a lower priority. It is important to maintain flexibility in response to both the student's and the preceptor's needs and preferences.

Strategies for Minimizing Costs

Primary care physicians are experiencing increasing pressure in their clinical practices. Compensation for additional time spent and for financial losses due to precepting has become more common and more financially important. As training for medical students shifts to the ambulatory arena, medical schools and legislators need to address compensation concerns. The benefits of teaching balance the costs of time and money. To keep this cost-benefit ratio favorable, preceptors are encouraged to review the following strategies and explore which ones may be applicable to their clinic, precepting style, and individual student.

Rewards and Reimbursement

- Monetary reimbursement may be available through medical school stipends.
- Encourage legislators to shift federal funds from the inpatient environment to support ambulatory teaching (Fields et al., 1998).
- Solicit local hospitals to support preceptor stipends and student room and board.
- Encourage medical schools to provide nonmonetary rewards. These typically include academic appointments, certificates, continuing medical education (CME) credit, access to library resources, training,

access to computer-based information sources such as
MEDLINE, travel to educational meetings, reduced
CME fees, and materials such as medical books or
journals.

Student Orientation and Initial Assessment

- Orient the student to the clinic and clinic personnel
  thoroughly and early. Provide a clear, written schedule. Use clinic staff to help orient and answer student
  questions.
- Assess an individual student's current skills and
  background before starting. Use this information to
  guide learning opportunities.
- Ask students about their learning style (e.g., cognitive,
  action) and adjust your teaching accordingly.

Scheduling

- Arrive at clinic early. Review schedule ahead of time
  to familiarize yourself with patient charts and choose
  with the student the patients it will be beneficial for
  them to see.
- Consider blocking out some patient slots from your
  schedule for catch-up and teaching.
- Students will use an exam room longer. Try to have
  extra exam rooms available if possible. Students do
  excellent histories and physicals. Use these skills with
  patients who need a longer interview. You can see
  other acute patients during this period.
- Experiment and be creative with nontraditional
  schedule designs.
  - Use a "wave" schedule. In this system, preceptor
    and student each start seeing patients at the
    beginning of each wave, and thereafter overlap at
    some point in the wave (Ferenchick et al., 1997).
  - Schedule many short or acute-care visits back to

back. Preceptor and student each see patients, depending on the length of the visit.
- Alternate patients (or entire clinics) between preceptor and student. Teacher and learner each take turns observing the other's entire patient encounters.

■ Invite the student to give a presentation and designate an occasional half day from the clinic for preparation. Include nonphysician staff in the audience because they may benefit from this medical education opportunity, a nonmonetary reward for the extra time they spend with students.

■ Share teaching responsibilities. Rotate primary precepting responsibilities among colleagues. Schedule the student with clinic staff to learn specific skills (e.g., administration of injections, telephone triage, performance of lab tests).

■ Consider increasing the number of students precepted per year. The more frequently a physician precepts a student, the less significant the impact on their practice (Bell and Frey, 1998).

■ In our experience, extending the length of a rotation helps any losses in productivity early in the course to be outweighed by later gains.

Structuring the Patient Encounter

■ Before the student sees a patient:
- Set specific goals for student participation.
- Review the differential diagnoses of the patient's chief complaint and appropriate questions the student might ask the patient.
- Give direction about time expectations.
- Request that after the time allotment, the student present to the preceptor a two- to three-minute focused presentation of findings.

- Maximize teaching in the examining room, educating both student and patient. This technique avoids repetition and provides rich material for direct observation, supervision, and feedback. Students are provided with role modeling and one-on-one teaching time with their preceptor. Patients appreciate it.
- Rather than waiting until the entire patient encounter is completed, a preceptor can enter the patient room after the student has performed the history and physical. The student presents the case in front of the patient. Student and preceptor then finish the evaluation together, ask the patient any remaining questions, and complete any remaining physical exam. At that point, the preceptor can gauge for each case whether the diagnosis and plan can be discussed in the presence of the patient or is more appropriately discussed outside the patient's room. To the extent possible, try to do this in the room with the patient present.
- Plan to directly observe a student's entire patient encounter. Particularly with time-intensive visits (e.g., annual exam or well-child check), direct observation eliminates the need for the student to present the entire history and exam to the preceptor.
- Discuss only issues important to the diagnosis and treatment at the time of the visit.

Effective and Efficient Teaching Strategies

- Encourage active, self-directed learning. "If you find yourself giving many mini-lectures on medical topics, you are still using a passive learning model and slowing down your clinical practice" (Scherger and Usatine, 1996). Ask students to develop a list of learning goals they especially want to pursue during the rotation. Encourage students to look up information in books, journals, and on the Internet and

MEDLINE. Occasionally ask the student to review the entire clinic schedule and take the initiative to plan their own schedule around interesting problems and procedures.

■ Delegate. If students check test results, call consultants, or write out prescriptions, they will learn from these tasks.

■ Use instructional videos (e.g., for a pelvic exam, infection control) and computerized patient management problems, especially for students early in their training. These are usually available through the medical school.

■ Maximize opportunities to incorporate teaching tasks (e.g., orientation or feedback) into other activities, such as a staff meeting or breakfast meeting.

■ Allow inexperienced students to initially observe rather than participate, especially with focused exams and procedures (e.g., well-child exam, suturing, or casting).

■ Cash in on key teaching opportunities. Often these require a small effort on your part but carry big learning impact for students. For example, encourage students to attend births and family conferences.

■ Bring clinic schedulers into the loop. If they appreciate how important it is for a student to learn continuity of care, they can help facilitate the experience necessary for learning.

■ Stick to specifics about the current patient. Avoid extensive theorizing or sharing too many personal case reports.

■ Make one teaching point per patient. That way both you and your student are not overwhelmed (Baldwin, 1997).

■ Prepare students to work efficiently. Students need to learn how to accommodate their own practice style and incorporate sound time management. Give specific instruction and feedback. Midway through the rotation, have students evaluate their own time management and develop goals and strategies to work on during the last half of the rotation. Discuss styles of practice and how they relate to management of time and money. Use the student's successes and frustrations in clinic as case studies for discussion and problem solving.

■ Reframe all daily tasks as potential teaching tools. Handling an unexpected phone call provides the student a chance to learn either efficiency or empathetic listening. Dictating between patients instead of expanding on the differential diagnosis of anemia suggests that efficiency at the expense of something else is sometimes okay. Discussing a nonmedical topic over lunch offers a lesson on preventing burnout.

Preceptor Training and Self-Evaluation

■ Gain training in teaching skills and how to integrate students into busy practices. Learn the skills of time-limited precepting. Many medical schools have resources available for their preceptors.

■ Make precepting of students an agenda item at clinic staff meetings. Learn from your physician and nonphysician colleagues how they manage their time and revenue.

■ Evaluate your own style. Use this awareness to practice flexibility in picking and choosing time investments carefully. Be cognizant of your own needs as a preceptor as well as those of students. There are many ways for students to learn.

■ Ask colleagues how they save time teaching students.

■ Think long term. Your precepting is needed. Don't burn out.

References

Baldwin, L. M. 1997. Managing clinic time while precepting medical students. *Family Medicine* 29(1):13.

Bell, J., and Frey, D. 1998. Survey shows impact of students in preceptors' offices. Letter. *Family Medicine* 30(2):82.

Ferenchick, G., Simpson, D., Blackman, J., DaRosa, D., and Dunnington, G. 1997. Strategies for efficient and effective teaching in the ambulatory care setting. *Academic Medicine* 72(4):277–80.

Fields, S. A., Usatine, R., Stearns, J. A., Toffler, W. L., and Vinson, D. C. 1998. The use and compensation of community preceptors in U.S. medical schools. *Academic Medicine* 73:95–97.

Ricer, R. E., Filak, A. T., and David, A. K. 1998. Determining the costs of a required third-year family medicine clerkship in an ambulatory setting. *Academic Medicine* 73(7):809–11.

Ricer, R. E., Van Horne, A., and Filak, A. T. 1997. Costs of preceptors' time spent teaching during a third-year family medicine outpatient rotation. *Academic Medicine* 72(6):547–51.

Scherger, J. E., and Usatine, R. P. 1996. Tips for preceptors who teach medical students in managed care settings. *Family Medicine* 28(10):688–89.

Logistics

Cheryl A. Abboud, M.P.A.

Key Points

- Medical students precepting in your office may require logistical support, including room and board.
- Your local hospital may be able to provide students with room and board.
- Written materials that describe your site logistics will be invaluable for students precepting in your office.

The decision to precept medical students, especially for an extended period of time, requires the consideration of many practical tasks. Room and board, food, mileage reimbursement, and other logistics must be arranged before the beginning of a rotation in order to ensure a successful experience for all.

Unless they are commuting to and from the site, students will almost always require housing while on their rotation. It is usually the responsibility of the site to arrange and pay for the housing costs. Assigning this responsibility to one person (e.g., the office manager or hospital administrator) will help ensure that all arrangements are taken care of consistently. There are several options for student accommodations. A hospital-owned apartment or house, a motel room, a hospital room, or a private home are most commonly used. The choice of the best alternative depends on the situation. For example, many hospitals own a small apartment or house used specifically for students and other out-of-town guests (e.g., residents). Check with your hospital administrator to see if this is available; if it is not, determine the likelihood of arranging permanent housing in the future.

Although the purchase of a small house may seem like a large initial investment, sites that have students year-round find this approach is less costly (and time-consuming) than trying to arrange housing on an individual basis throughout the year. A selling point to the hospital could be that the house may be used for students of all types: nursing, pharmacy, and physician assistants, as well as medical students. Another selling point may be the issue of recruiting future health care providers into the community. Having students spend time in a community is a great opportunity to recruit future practitioners, and adequate housing always enhances the chances of students choosing a site for a rotation. If the community elects to purchase a house for students to use while on rotation, an important consideration is location. Close proximity to the clinic and hospital is beneficial, allowing students quick access for on-call or emergency situations. Your site may also want to consider supplying students with a pager for emergency cases.

If a permanent house or apartment is not possible, there are several other alternatives. Many hospitals have one or more rooms converted into dormitory-type accommodations. Although this arrangement may not provide all the amenities of a home, it can provide the student with needed space and privacy. Some communities opt to have students stay with a member of the clinic or a volunteer from the community. This is definitely less expensive for the site, but space and privacy become a prime concern. If you choose this option, it is extremely important that the parties understand the "rules," such as which parts of the house the student will have access to and when "quiet" time is in effect. Regardless of the type of accommodation, it is essential to inform your student about what is required. Many students do not think to bring their own linens or cooking utensils. Giving the student a list of recommended items helps to ensure a comfortable experience. You may also want to inform the student about the availability of laundry facilities, phone service, and local attractions.

Not all students rotating in your community require housing. Some students select certain communities because family members live in or near the town, and in such instances they may choose to stay with family. It never hurts to ask whether accommodations will be needed.

Many sites provide students with a meal ticket good for breakfast, lunch, and dinner at the hospital. Students are thus given the chance for a free meal when it is needed or wanted. Other communities simply provide the student with an employee discount at the hospital cafeteria. Either of these options is satisfactory, and making one or the other available is especially important if students are staying in a hospital room, motel room, or other type of housing where cooking is not possible. When provided with this courtesy, students usually understand that if they choose to eat elsewhere in the community, they do so at their own expense. For those communities that provide students with an apartment or house, basic items such as sugar, salt, and other staples, as well as some toiletry items, are often supplied. If students need to bring or replace any items, they should be informed of this fact before the start of the rotation.

Many universities ask their community sites to provide the students with one round-trip mileage reimbursement to and from the site at the Internal Revenue Service mileage rate. If it is not possible for your site to reimburse the student for this expense, informing the student of this decision up-front can avoid an awkward situation at the end of the rotation. Some communities also have students spend a day or two a week traveling to satellite clinics in neighboring communities. Again, reimbursement for mileage should be considered if such travel is a requirement of the rotation.

As more and more hospitals become involved in the clinician's practice, many of these hospitals are requiring contracts or affiliation agreements with the partnering university. The coordinators for the university's various departments (e.g., family medicine, internal medicine, pediatrics, or the dean's business office) should be able to provide you with the information needed for formulating an affiliation agreement. The responsibilities of the university and the community site in safeguarding the students against medical hazards should be a primary issue addressed in this agreement. Malpractice insurance, immunization records, and adherence to federal, state, and local regulations, such as the Americans with Disabilities Act (ADA), should also be documented. A more informal guide to expectations is often available through individual departments of the university. Asking the various departments for a copy of their preceptor guidelines will provide you with general recommendations to follow regarding the teaching and supervision of your students.

Another expense a site may encounter when precepting medical students is the payment of a stipend. Although a stipend is not always required, many preceptors feel students have provided enough help to justify payment for their service. Whether a stipend is required by the university should be stated in the university's preceptor guidelines. If this is a requirement or recommendation for the rotation, you may want to turn to your hospital administrator for assistance with this cost.

A few other expenses come with the precepting of students, including long-distance phone charges, cable TV service, and cleanup and maintenance of the housing unit. Charges that will be the responsibility of the student should be discussed during the student's orientation.

Having students precept at your clinic can be a rewarding and enjoyable experience for both the preceptor and preceptee. Coordination is essential, however, to ensuring that excessive time is not spent sorting out financial and logistical issues. Communication between your office staff and the university's coordinating staff can do much to improve the precepting experience for all. Providing a short flyer outlining your room, board, reimbursement, and other policies which can be sent to students in advance of the rotation can alleviate many problems and enhance the rotation. Assigning one central contact person at the site to take care of details beforehand will enable the preceptor to spend quality time with his or her students, teaching, mentoring, and learning.

■ 24

Involving Your Office Staff in Teaching

Curtis C. Stine, M.D., and Roger C. Shenkel, M.D.

Key Points

The essentials of involving your office staff in teaching medical students are:

- Maintain an office environment where staff members have defined roles, work well together as a team, and are valued by the physician.
- Communicate with staff members before the student's arrival.
- Introduce the student to each staff member very early in the rotation and involve appropriate office staff members in the student's orientation.
- Schedule time during the rotation for the student and key staff members to discuss each staff member's role and responsibilities in greater detail.
- Involve staff members in identifying patients who agree to be seen by the student.

Community-based preceptorships and clerkships typically occur in physician's offices, residency training practices, or other free-standing clinics. These community-based experiences expose students to the structure and operation of a "real" physician office and to staff members who assist the physician-preceptor. In addition, these rotations may be the student's sole exposure to common practice management issues. Staff members can contribute to the student's education, and the preceptor should seek to involve them in the student experience.

The individual staff member's ability to meaningfully

contribute to the student preceptorship is enhanced when staff roles and responsibilities have been clearly defined and when staff members function together as a team. Furthermore, staff members must feel valued for their personal contributions, and understand their unique role in the successful operation of the practice.

The office staff should be informed of the student rotation well in advance of the student's arrival. This advance notice allows them to make any necessary adjustments in the patient schedule and to prepare essential student materials.

On the day the student arrives, the physician-preceptor should introduce the student to each member of the office team and describe each team member's responsibility. Name tags for both the student and the office staff can facilitate the memorization of names and titles. It is often appropriate to involve key staff members in other aspects of the student's orientation. For example, it is completely appropriate to allow the nurse or medical assistant to orient the student to the layout of each room, or permit the fee coordinator to orient the student to billing and coding obligations. In addition, the student should become familiar with the organization of the medical record system. If the student is required to dictate items for the medical record, the transcriptionist should instruct the student in dictation and transcription protocol. If the rotation requires the student to complete a project, identify the materials and data needed and, if appropriate, the staff member who will assist the student.

During the student's orientation, an appropriate block of time may be scheduled later in the rotation with each key staff member. During these scheduled times, the student will directly observe staff members performing their jobs. Scheduling the blocks in advance permits staff members to avoid busy days or busy times in the office and to prepare any documents or handouts for the student ses-

Table 24.1. ■ Potential educational topics to be taught by office staff members

Office Staff Member	Topic
Nurse or medical assistant	Orienting to layout of exam rooms
	Taking vital signs
	Giving injections
Laboratory technician	Venipuncture and drawing blood
	Performing office-based lab tests
	Reviewing or reporting lab results
X-ray technician	Positioning patients for X-rays
	Processing X-rays
Receptionist	Answering the telephone
	Making appointments
	Greeting patients and updating information
	Explaining billing policies
Check-out person	Ensuring completeness of billing forms
	Requesting payments on account
	Arranging follow-up appointments
Transcriptionist	Using dictation equipment
	Transcription etiquette and protocol
	Common transcription errors
Office manager	Overview of financial policies
	Overview of personnel policies
	Review of practice financial data
	Special practice contracts and agreements

sion. As key staff members meet with the student, have them describe their specific tasks and roles. Allow the staff members to determine additional educational topics. Examples of appropriate educational content taught by identified office staff members are included in Table 24.1. Encourage staff members to answer student questions. Invite the student to participate in all office staff meetings. Remind staff members who are reluctant or uncomfortable in a teaching role that they have expertise to share with the students in a unique learning environment.

Certain office staff members have a critical role in further introducing the student to patients. As patients register, the receptionist or medical office assistant should inform the patient that a medical student is working with the physician and inquire whether the patient has any objections to being seen by the student. If a patient objects, the receptionist should notify the nurse or medical assistant of the patient's concerns. When patients agree to be seen by the student, the nurse or medical assistant should inform them of the student's name. When necessary, they should reassure the patient that the physician will also see them and supervise all medical decisions.

As the rotation is ending, solicit specific feedback from office staff members to include in the student's final evaluation. If the student has completed a project during the rotation, invite the student to present the project results to the entire office staff. Commemorate the end of the student rotation with an office staff activity, allowing the staff and the student to say good-bye.

Relationships to Medical Schools and Other Agencies

Working with Preceptorship Sponsors: Medical Schools and Clinical Departments

Katherine C. Krause, M.D., James MacColl Nicholson, M.D., and Patrick T. Waters, D.O.

Key Points
- Medical schools and departments of family medicine should support preceptors as they learn about incentives to teach and opportunities to improve their skills.
- Preceptors should be proactive and make sure that they understand the goals and objectives of the preceptorship experience, the level of the student's training, and expectations regarding evaluation.
- Preceptors should get feedback on their teaching.

When you teach medical students in your office, you will interact with the students' sponsoring school and departments. The following information and advice will assist you in these interactions.
- Ask what the school is prepared to do to diagnose and remediate a challenging learner who is assigned to your practice: one who doesn't want to be there, has a learning difficulty, or is having personal problems (Chapter 19).
- Ask about the incentives to teach. Although they may not be financial, they may have considerable value: precepting students may be counted as part of your production; you may also receive computer equipment and training, medical textbooks, teaching heads for microscopes or ophthalmoscopes, online connections to the library, diagnostic data banks, patient

education printouts, e-mail, free continuing medical
education, and faculty development programs.

- At a minimum, ask for goals and objectives, a course
  outline and schedule, evaluation forms, a textbook or
  list of readings, and a set of supervisory expectations.
  Some programs will send you a special preceptor's
  teaching manual.
- Choose a point person in your practice who will act as
  a contact for the medical school, and ask the sponsoring program to choose a similar person with whom
  you can communicate directly.
- Tell both the department and the medical school how
  best to communicate with you and your students. Do
  you prefer phone, fax, e-mail, or regular mail? What
  level of computer expertise and equipment is expected?
- If the medical school or department does not use
  formal learning contracts to provide information on
  the student's background, experience, and personal
  goals for the rotation, ask each student to give you
  these goals so you can set mutual expectations for the
  rotation (see Chapter 12).
- Identify your most effective advocate in the department of family medicine; this is usually the predoctoral education director. In the dean's office it may be
  the coordinator of the primary care network. Both
  have experience with almost any situation you can
  anticipate and are paid to be problem solvers; use
  them and their resources. Have them visit your
  practice and observe you and your students in action
  so their tips will be practical.
- Ask the family medicine department if they have a
  preceptor advisory board to provide feedback on the
  medical student curriculum. Call them for advice.
- Find out from the department what faculty appointments are offered for what degree of commitment to

the teaching mission. Is there an organized plan for promotion?

- Return student evaluation forms expeditiously so you can provide focused, behaviorally linked feedback. Encourage your school to attach behavioral descriptors to the grades to aid you in assessing student performance. Give examples from specific patient-student encounters.
- Ask that the institution or department provide you with student evaluations of your practice.
- How do the institution and the department emphasize the importance and role of a community-based practice experience as part of the medical school curriculum before their students come to your office?

■ **26**

Preparing for a Site Visit

James L. Brand, M.D., and
JoAnn M. Carpenter, M.D.

Key Points

- Site visits are an important part of communication between the preceptor's site and the sponsoring institution.
- Areas of review during a site visit usually include supervision, the office and other teaching environments, housing, meals and support services, library and other educational resources, and balance between patient care and free time.
- The site visit provides the opportunity to outline the strengths and weaknesses of the preceptorship program and strategies for improvement.

Site visits are an integral part of the development and maintenance of preceptorships. This chapter assists the community preceptor in preparing for a successful site review. During these visits, whether for developing a new site or visiting an established one, a course director will review a variety of aspects integral to student education to ensure that the educational goals established by the college of medicine are met. This process includes a review of not only the patient care experience but also the environment in which the student learns. Urban and rural sites are similar in respect to preceptor qualification, office and library milieu, and community involvement. They may differ in the areas of student housing and night supervision. In general, the areas reviewed during a site visit should include but not be limited to:

142

- supervision
- community involvement
- office
- free time
- housing and meals
- continuing medical education
- library
- safety
- patient contact

Overview of the Visit

Site visits will generally occur every three to five years, but they may take place sooner if new preceptors are added to the site, if students have identified issues that are difficult to resolve, or if the visits are requested by the preceptor. Preceptors should feel free to request site visits by the course director(s). Most preceptors donate their time to their respective medical school and therefore should be afforded the courtesy of a site visit scheduled at their convenience. Scheduled visits allow the preceptor time to arrange a meeting with the administrator(s) of the health care facilities and nursing supervisors. Meeting the administrative staff allows the course director an opportunity to convey the college of medicine's gratitude to all the professionals involved in educating medical students. The total site visit usually requires no more than three hours.

Supervision

Supervision is perhaps the most important item to be reviewed. The preceptor should be prepared to outline the system used to supervise the student in the outpatient and inpatient settings. There should also be a discussion of student supervision during evenings, weekends, and holidays.

Emergency department (ED) responsibilities require specific discussion regarding supervision. If the student evaluates patients in the ED, regardless of the time of day, clear lines of supervision should be outlined. Several questions need to be specifically addressed with the reviewer:

- If a full-time provider staffs the ED, has that provider agreed to supervise the student?
- In EDs where no full-time staff is present, who determines if the student evaluates the patient?
- If the student evaluates the patient, when does the student discuss the patient with the preceptor: before or after the history or the exam, prior to ordering tests or medications, or only if admission is necessary?

Supervision requirements vary from college to college. Generally, colleges reinforce supervisory issues related to state licensure. Ideally, supervision would occur during the entire student-patient encounter, but this can be stifling and interfere with student-patient rapport. Students should review the patient with the preceptor early in the course of care, after the history or initial exam, but before any treatment, testing, or medication is initiated.

The documentation of student supervision is important, not only from the medical-legal standpoint but also with regard to billing issues. Health Care Financing Administration (HCFA) guidelines do not require the teaching physician to redocument the review of systems and past, family, and social history *if* they are well documented by the student in a written or dictated note. However, the teaching physician *must* perform and briefly restate the history of the present illness. The HCFA rules state that the teaching physician must perform the physical exam and document the key elements in order to bill a fee (memorandum from R. Dickler, Division of Health Care Affairs, Association of American Medical Colleges, Feb. 3, 1997).

Office

A site visit must include a review of ambulatory care areas. The reviewer should visit the office waiting area and exam rooms. This portion of the site review will focus on the reference library; Internet access; patient record-keeping; and available laboratory, radiology, and ancillary services.

The educational objectives at ambulatory sites may be best achieved if the student encounters a representative sample of patients (Kennedy, 1980). This is why the demographics of the practice should be discussed. The mix of private pay, third-party payer, Medicare, Medicaid, and managed care patients should be discussed to assist the reviewer in developing an overall view of the practice. The demographics of a community practice may be different from those in ambulatory care centers at academic health centers.

The method of record-keeping (written, transcribed, standardized forms) should be reviewed for completeness, legibility, and the system of filing loose paperwork. This is as important as the review of patient care experiences, since adequate and appropriate record-keeping habits will have a significant impact on the student's lifelong professional practice.

Continuing Medical Education

Generally, preceptors are required to maintain current specialty board certification. The preceptor's certification status may be reviewed during the site visit. Many specialty boards reward preceptors for their teaching efforts with continuing medical education (CME) credit.

General Considerations

Housing and Meals

Rural preceptorships may be established in a community located at a distance from the main academic campus. This often requires the sponsoring practice or hospital to provide for student housing (Brand, 1997). Some colleges require the student to cover the housing expense, which may be tied to a stipend provided by an academic or government-sponsored program (Verby, 1977). Options for housing include a former patient room or an off-campus site such as a motel room, apartment, or house. Student quarters should be distant from active patient care to allow the student both privacy and a quiet sleeping area. Meals are often a benefit given the student, typically at the hospital cafeteria.

Safety

Students frequently identify safety concerns when completing postclerkship evaluations. Whether in-hospital or offsite, student housing must include a telephone, adequate lighting between the parking area and the housing entrance, and a functioning fire alarm (Brand, 1997).

Library or Online Service

The college, as a standard part of a preceptorship, should offer access to information resources, photocopying, and library services for the practice at no charge or at a reduced fee. Many colleges offer Internet or e-mail access.

Free Time

Adequate free time is important to the morale of the student and sometimes the preceptor. This time offers students an opportunity to return to their homes and families, collect their mail, and pay bills.

Call Schedule

The call schedule should be available for review to ensure that a system is in place for student supervision. This document is most important in settings where students are more often the first responders to emergency department calls and urgent inpatient needs. A night-call system ensures that the student will not be up every night addressing ED or urgent inpatient needs. Failure to define nights off call may result in the student rarely getting a full night's sleep. This may lead to errors in judgment and dissatisfaction by the student and may put a given site at risk of being closed by the college of medicine. Students are generally on call no more than every third night.

Managed Health Care

Managed health care is more likely to be a part of an urban than a rural practice. Exposure to a managed health care organization has become more important to student education in the past decade. The student must be given the opportunity to learn how such organizations affect patient access to specialists, generic and brand-name pharmaceuticals, choice of hospitals, and primary care providers.

Departmental Functions

Many departments require the student to attend teaching conferences, grand rounds, or some other form of didactic session, all of which vary in format and time requirements. Although the preceptor may view the student's absence from the clinical practice site as an inconvenience, such sessions remind the student that continuing education will require regular participation in a formal setting.

Site Visit Wrap-Up

The end of the site visit period is a time to offer suggestions for improvement and to discuss areas of concern.

These discussions may focus on changes that will help a given practice or the preceptorship program in general. Preceptors describe the teaching of medical students as a positive experience and a stimulus for remaining current with the medical literature (Barritt et al., 1997).

The wrap-up is an opportunity for the course director to update preceptors on new college of medicine policies. These policies may affect all courses in general or the preceptorship specifically. It is also a chance for the preceptor to offer input on any changes that directly affect the preceptor and the teaching site. Thus, all aspects of a preceptorship program should be open for general discussion with the course director. Through these discussions the preceptor and the course director can work jointly for continued improvement of the preceptorship program.

References

Barritt, A., Silagy, C., Worley, P., Watts, R., Marley, J., and Gill, D. 1997. Attitudes of rural general practitioners toward undergraduate medical student attachments. *Australian Family Physician* 26 (Suppl. 2):S87–S90.

Brand, J. 1997. When your practice is under the microscope: how to survive a rural preceptorship site visit. *Family Medicine* 29(7):461–62.

Kennedy, V. C. 1980. Exposure to a rural population in a rural residency training program. *Journal of Community Health* 5(4):261–69.

Verby, J. 1977. The Minnesota rural physician redistribution plan, 1971–1976. *Journal of the American Medical Association* 238(9):960–64.

■ 27

Working with Area Health Education Centers

Joseph Hobbs, M.D.

Key Point

■ Area health education centers may help coordinate preceptorships, provide faculty development, and facilitate networking.

The increased emphasis on primary care education has required additional faculty, patient resources, and teaching sites beyond the traditional medical center boundaries. Many academic health science universities have developed primary care clinical programs in partnership with area health education centers (AHECs). These federally funded agencies can be a resource for the community preceptor in several areas.

Benefits of Working with AHECs

Student Scheduling

Some authorities feel that preceptors who teach students throughout the year incur lower teaching costs per student than preceptors who have students intermittently (Chapter 22). The AHECs often work with more than one medical school and may allow the preceptor a continuous supply of students as well as students at different training levels and from different backgrounds.

Coordination

Many AHEC directors can broker partnerships between the teaching site and the medical schools, facilitate stu-

149

dent acclimation to communities, and ensure student participation in nonacademic educational activities.

Faculty Development

AHECs can serve as a direct resource for faculty development or as a clearinghouse for faculty development resources.

Information

AHECs have explored the development of information networks for community preceptors, including access to medical information databases, the Internet, and other forms of information sharing.

Networking

AHECs often work with several teaching sites in a given area. They can facilitate the sharing of information, teaching concerns, and educational resources among preceptors across sites.

Working with Other Health Disciplines

AHECs work with health profession schools in a variety of disciplines. They may be able to coordinate rotations for students in nursing, pharmacy, and physician assistant training programs.

Financial Assistance

Some AHECs are able to assist students with room and board costs during community rotations. AHECs may also be able to assist community practice sites in obtaining the technology necessary for improving access to information.

General Support

AHECs can serve as information sources to solve educational and logistic problems, either directly or by helping the preceptor contact the appropriate person or agency. Because AHECs work with medical science universities, communities, and community teaching sites, they offer unique resources to the preceptor. AHECs can help improve your precepting. The national AHEC office can be contacted at:

Area Health Education Center
Department of Health and Human Services
Division of Medicine, Room 9A27, Parklawn Building
5600 Fishers Lane
Rockville, Md. 20857
(301) 443-6950

Working with Local Hospital Administrators

Joyce Copeland, M.D., Susan Epstein, M.P.A.,
Harold Krueger, and Gayle Primrose

Key Points

- Hosting a student provides tangible benefits to your local hospital and may enhance the recruitment and retention of physicians.
- Be clear about the services your local hospital will provide for visiting students.
- The sponsoring institution should help support you and your hospital.

Introducing students to the hospital environment represents an opportunity to model the role of the community physician in patient care. A community preceptor must consider the many roles and responsibilities of the hospital and its administrators when bringing a medical student into this setting.

Hospitals are frequently one of the largest employers in the community. Their financial viability and the quality of care they provide may have a direct impact on the fiscal health of the community. The reputation of the hospital and the community's perception of the quality of care are also critical. Hospital administrators and trustees are usually selected in part because they are fiscally and politically adept. Administrators walk a line between the will of the trustees and the desires of the medical staff. They balance the needs for technology, human resources, space, and equipment with the demand for sound economic policy. This task must be accomplished while maintaining the integrity of the hospital's mission in the community. Adding a student to this mixture of competing interests requires preparation and consideration of the impact of the student on the institution. Hospital administrators are obligated to justify the use of the hospital facilities for the education of the student while protecting the facility against liability. A wise administrator will also be looking for the advantages that the student may provide for the reputation and future of the facility.

The preceptor may be involved in medical, administrative, educational, and political activities within the hospital. Therefore, the preceptor should lay the necessary groundwork with the hospital administration, key medical colleagues, and hospital staff before bringing the student into the picture. If the preceptor does this far in advance of the first student's arrival, the administration and medical and hospital staff will know what to expect from the student's experience and what the student will expect from them. This groundwork should help the hospital administration and staff perceive the student as an asset. Note that to ensure proper insurance coverage, hospitals need to inform their malpractice carriers that this educational program will be conducted within the facility.

What Are the Potential Benefits to the Hospital and Community of Teaching Medical Students?

Medical students are potential recruits to the local medical staff and community and offer the hospital an opportunity to:

- preview the skills and interests of the student
- market the community and hospital to the student
- create a potential ambassador for the community through networking with the student and the academic medical center
- build and sustain a tie between the hospital and the academic medical center

- enhance the reputation of the hospital as an institution of a quality that supports medical education

The hospital can support the teaching efforts of the medical staff. This support can provide intangible rewards by (Gerrity et al., 1997; Grayson et al., 1998; Pathman, 1993):

- enhancing satisfaction of the preceptor who teaches and serves as role model
- sharpening the skills of the preceptor who is being observed and challenged by the responsibility for teaching
- expanding the skills of the hospital staff through exposure to new and current medical trends
- engaging in the tradition of the medical apprenticeship by developing future physicians
- improving the retention of physicians for the community
- enriching the experience of the patients by the attention they receive from the student and the feeling that they are contributing to the student's education (York et al., 1995)
- enriching the professional role of the hospital staff who work with and teach students about their function on the care team

What Are the Potential Liabilities of Having a Student in the Hospital?

Potential liabilities include:

- the presence of an unlicensed caregiver with access to patients and data
- uncertainty regarding the clinical and interpersonal skills of the student
- possible change in hospital routine
- liability for the care of the patients and thus concerns for risk management

How Can the Preceptor Persuade the Hospital to Accept Students?

The preceptor can:
- ensure and provide active and visible supervision of the student
- clarify the role of the student and the limitations of the student's authority with the hospital administrator, medical colleagues, and hospital staff
- introduce the student to key administrators, medical colleagues, and hospital staff
- prepare the student for the hospital experience:
  - hospital policy
  - duties and limitations
  - role and responsibilities of the community physician in the hospital
- encourage the student to participate in service activities that benefit the community
- insist on professional appearance and personal behavior

What Services Might the Local Hospital Provide for the Medical Student?

The local hospital may provide:
- housing (students should inform the hospital if they have any special needs, are bringing a spouse, family, dog, etc.)
- meals (students should inform the hospital if they have any special diet needs, restrictions, etc.)
- parking
- library services
- telephone, fax, copying services
- access to the Internet
- community memberships (e.g., fitness center)

What Should the Preceptor and Hospital Expect from the Medical School?

The medical school should provide:

- training for the student in prevention of respiratory and blood-borne pathogens with appropriate documentation
- documentation of the student's immunizations if requested
- clarification and documentation of the responsibility for health coverage for the student
- education of the student about professional ethics, demeanor, and responsibility for intervention should problems be identified
- availability and visibility of a course director who is responsible for the curriculum and for troubleshooting when the need arises
- documentation of liability coverage for the student's activities during the rotation; this information should be sent to the hospital before the student arrives so that any questions or concerns can be addressed before the start of the educational rotation

Who Can Help the Preceptor with this Process?

Regional area health education centers may have already established a teaching agreement with the hospital. If not, they might be willing to help or take responsibility for the process. The hospital may have a person or department responsible for educational activities in the facility.

Acknowledgments

Thanks to the following for input on the role of area health education centers: Debbie Fisher, Charlotte, North Carolina, AHEC, Office of Regional Primary Care Education, and Katherine McGinnis, Eastern Area Health Education Center, Office of Regional Primary Care Education.

References

Gerrity, M., Pathman, D., Linzer, M., Steiner, B., Winterbottom, L., Sharp, M., and Skochelak, S. 1997. Career satisfaction and clinician-educators. *Journal of General Internal Medicine* 12:S90–S97.

Grayson, M., Lein, M., Lugo, J., and Visintainer, P. 1998. Benefits and costs to community-based physicians teaching primary care to medical students. *Journal of General Internal Medicine* 13(7):485–88.

Pathman, D. 1993. Recruitment and retention of physicians in HPSAS presented at practice sites. State primary care development strategies technical assistance workshop. Asheville, N.C.

York, N., DaRosa, D., Markwell, S., Neihaus, A., and Folse, R. 1995. Patients' attitudes toward the involvement of medical students in their care. *American Journal of Surgery* 169(4):421–23.

▪ 29

Preceptors in Managed Care Organizations

Richard P. Usatine, M.D., and
Joseph E. Scherger, M.D., M.P.H.

Key Points

Preceptors in managed care settings can deal effectively with the time demands of precepting by:
- setting clear goals for students
- giving direction about time expectations
- giving students responsibility appropriate to their level of learning
- promoting active learning and contributions to patient care
- giving regular and specific feedback

Managed care organizations are becoming more common payers for health services and may encourage physicians to precept medical students or discourage them from doing so. As market forces continue to promote increasing numbers of managed care arrangements, students will need to graduate from medical school having had practice experience in managed care settings. Primary care physicians working in managed care settings are an important resource for teaching medical students this style of practice (Usatine et al., 1997).

Managed care organizations may be interested in having their primary care physicians precept medical students if they believe this activity will enhance the quality of patient care. Also, medical students may contribute to patient care by providing additional communication and patient education. Managed care organizations will not want their primary care physicians precepting if this activity reduces physicians' productivity and interferes with patient flow. Hence, primary care physicians in managed care organizations should focus on having the medical students add value to patient care sessions without reducing productivity.

The following strategies are suggested to help preceptors in managed care settings deal effectively with the time pressures of precepting students in a fast-paced ambulatory environment:

- Set specific goals for student participation.
- Give the student direction about time expectations.
- Give the student increasing levels of responsibility as you assess their skill level.
- Promote active learning by the student.
- Help the student contribute productively to caring for patients.
- Give the student regular and specific feedback.

Set Specific Goals for Student Participation

Before sending a student to see a patient, examine the chart and chief complaint with the student and set a limited goal for the patient's visit. For example, if the chief complaint is low back pain, you may ask the student to do a focused history and physical exam related to back pain. Give your student guidance on what essential questions and physical exam maneuvers are expected for the presenting problem. Effective planning can clarify expectations for student performance, select patients appropriate to learner level and time available, and better enable students to conduct focused, time-efficient histories and physical exams (Ferenchick et al., 1997).

Give the Student Direction about Time Expectations

Giving direction about time expectations and teaching the student how to focus will help you, your patients, and your student manage time more efficiently. For example, suggest that the student spend 15 to 20 minutes performing a focused history and physical. Show the student how you make decisions about time allocation. Time-management skills are essential to all medical practice.

Give the Student Increasing Levels of Responsibility as You Assess Their Skill Level

Students want hands-on experience with patients. Give them brief preparatory information on the patient and then send them in to see patients independently (at least to conduct the history and initial physical exam, as their training allows). They should be encouraged to devise an assessment and plan, and they should be expected to complete the charting on their patients.

Once you're ready to join your patient and student, ask the student to present the case even if the exam has not been completed. Sometimes it may be appropriate to have the student present the case in front of the patient and then you and the student finish evaluating the patient together. Encourage the student to provide health education to a patient. For example, you may give the student a health education handout to review with the patient.

If you have the student observe what you are doing, consider performing an active demonstration in which you provide explanations before, during, and after the demonstration. This process transforms a passive learning situation into an active one.

Teach students and patients simultaneously. Explain disease processes, treatment plans, and health promotion to the patient while the student is in the exam room. This allows you to model good doctor-patient communication and health education while teaching both the patient and the student. This strategy avoids splitting your time and attention between patient and student.

Promote Active Learning by the Student

If you find yourself giving many mini-lectures on medical topics to your students, you are still using a passive learning model and slowing down your clinical practice. Encourage the student to look up information in books and journals and through the Internet and MEDLINE. You may point the student in the right direction, but don't do the work for them. The process of information retrieval and active learning is as important as the content to be learned.

Help the Student Contribute Productively to Caring for Patients

Students can add value to a preceptor's practice by helping with many aspects of providing care for patients (Scherger and Fowkes, 1997). With adequate student training in ambulatory care and informatics, students will be able to enhance your practice. Examples include having the student write notes in patient charts and provide health education to patients. Encourage the student to look up essential information about a patient's problem. This process may involve using online resources.

Give the Student Regular and Specific Feedback

Give regular and specific feedback to students on their histories, physical exams, presentations, charting, and clinical reasoning. When listening to a student's presen-

Table 29.1. ■ Clinical teaching microskills

Get a commitment	"What do you think is going on with this patient?"
	"What would you like to do next?"
	Determine the student's view of the case.
	Don't just ask for more data about the patient.
	Don't immediately provide the answer to the problem.
Probe for underlying reasoning	"What led you to that conclusion?"
	"What else did you consider and rule out?"
	Diagnose the learner's understanding of the case—gaps in knowledge, poor reasoning or attitudes, misunderstandings.
	Don't just ask for texbook knowledge.
Teach a general rule	"The key features of this illness are . . ."
	The teaching point should help the student generalize from this case to other cases.
Tell the learner what he or she did right	State specifically what was done well and why it is important. This should not be general praise; be specific.
Correct errors	"Next time this happens, try this . . ."
	Make recommendations for improvement; be future oriented. Uncorrected errors may be repeated.

Source: Adapted from J. Neher, C. Gordon, B. Meyer, and N. Stevens (1992), A five-step "microskills" model of clinical teaching, *American Board of Family Practice* 5:688–89.

tation of a case, use the microskills of the one-minute preceptor (get a commitment, probe for underlying reasoning, teach a general principle, provide positive feedback, and correct errors) (Neher et al., 1992). This can be initiated by two simple questions: "What do you think is going on? What led you to that conclusion?" These microskills allow the preceptor to diagnose the learner, teach general rules, and provide effective feedback (Table 29.1).

Allowing your student to see patients independently and write the chart notes will save time. It also gives you the opportunity to provide feedback on performance. Giving immediate feedback improves the learning experience.

The Role of the Managed Care Organization

What can managed care organizations do to support their preceptors? At a minimum, preceptors should be recognized and rewarded for this teaching. Access to online resources is also quite helpful in promoting evidence-based medicine and high-quality teaching. This teaching will benefit managed care organizations when these students are practicing in the future. It is also important to give preceptors extra time for teaching in their schedules.

In conclusion, medical education needs committed and trained preceptors in managed care settings who can be role models and mentors for medical students. As preceptors' teaching skills develop, they can practice efficiently with students. Medical schools and managed care organizations must support preceptors if we are to succeed in recruiting, training, and retaining skilled teachers.

References

Ferenchick, G., Simpson, D., Blackman, J., DaRosa, D., and Dunnington, G. 1997. Strategies for efficient and effective teaching in the ambulatory care setting. *Academic Medicine* 72:277–80.

Neher, J., Gordon, C., Meyer, B., and Stevens, N. 1992. A five-step "microskills" model of clinical teaching. *American Board of Family Practice* 5:688–89.

Scherger, J. E., and Fowkes, W. C. 1997. It's time to put medical students back to work (editorial). *Family Medicine* 29(2):137–38.

Usatine, R., Nguyen, K., Randall, J., and Irby, D. 1997. Four exemplary preceptors' strategies for efficient teaching in managed care settings. *Academic Medicine* 72 (9):766–69. Adapted in part from R. Usatine and J. Scherger (1996), Tips for preceptors teaching medical students in managed care settings, *Family Medicine* 28(10):688–89.

■ **VI**

Legal and Ethical Aspects of Precepting

▪ 30

Liability Issues for Preceptors

Richard G. Roberts, M.D., J.D.

Key Points
- The liability risks of serving as a preceptor are minimal.
- A well-informed patient and a professional demeanor protect against most risks.
- Professional liability insurance policies usually cover most risks related to teaching.

Few issues inflame the passions of physicians as readily as liability concerns. The fear of litigation can be paralyzing for some doctors and may be their stated reason for abstaining from certain activities that are perceived as high risk, such as maternity care (Roberts, Bobula, and Wolkomir, 1998). Some physicians may offer malpractice worries as their reason for not serving as preceptors. Such fears are often inappropriate or excessive, especially when one considers that the overall risk of a lawsuit is relatively low, about 1 in 40,000 patient encounters; the risk is even lower for teaching activities (Roberts, 1995). Put more bluntly, when doctors cite liability concerns as their reason for not participating as preceptors, it usually means that they are misinformed about the magnitude of risk associated with teaching or that they are searching for a more polite reason to decline participation. This chapter examines the nature of the liability risks associated with teaching and offers strategies for reducing those risks.

Agency and *Respondeat Superior*

Under the doctrine of *respondeat superior*, supervisors are held liable for the negligent acts of those who serve as their agents. The determination of whether agency and liability should apply in a specific case will turn on the degree of control exerted by the supervisor. In health care, the legal assumption is that attending physicians control and therefore remain ultimately responsible for the care provided to their patients. Thus, students and residents who participate in that care are said to do so as agents of and under the supervision of the attending doctor (Oliver, 1986). As a result, the physician's liability exposure resulting from the supervision of trainees is not substantially different than the risks posed by supervising other health care workers (e.g., medical assistants). It is, therefore, important for preceptors to know the abilities of their trainees and adjust the intensity of their supervision to fit the needs of the patient and the trainee.

Patient Consent

Most patients want to know who is involved in their care. Common courtesy would advise that every person who comes into direct contact with patients be introduced to them. The legal right of patients to choose who is involved in their care requires that they know the identity and status of the various team members. Although there is little risk in being sued for failure to inform a patient that a caregiver is a trainee (Kapp, 1983), introducing trainees and securing the permission of the patient for their participation should be a routine part of every patient encounter involving students and residents. Identification tags should provide the trainee's name and training status. Patient requests that certain trainees not be involved in their care should be respected.

Evaluation

Most physicians focus their liability concerns on suits filed by patients, but teaching physicians must also be aware of the potential for suits by learners. The evaluation of learners is inevitably a subjective process. However, training preceptors in the use of criterion-based evaluation reduces the chance of litigation from students who receive negative evaluations (Kapp, 1981). A criterion-based evaluation uses objective criteria, or standards, against which the learner's performance is measured (e.g., "all elements of the physical exam were performed properly").

Other Issues

Teachers must be ever mindful that they are in a status relationship with respect to learners. Status relationships involve a differential in power between two parties, such as teacher and learner or employer and employee. This inequity can leave the party with greater power subject to allegations of intimidation, sexual harassment, or other claims of impropriety if the relationship becomes inappropriate. Many universities have developed codes of faculty conduct to deal with these complex issues.

Liability Protection

In the unlikely event of a lawsuit, it is essential that a preceptor have liability coverage, such as a doctor's professional liability insurance policy. Most medical malpractice policies provide defense costs and indemnification for claims arising out of teaching activities. It is recognized that physicians who teach tend to stay more current in their medical knowledge and represent a lower overall liability risk. Thus, most insurance carriers are usually supportive of an insured's teaching activities. In addition, medical schools and residencies will often have insurance policies that provide coverage for teaching duties when the doctor's own insurance company does not. It should be noted that insurance policies do not provide coverage for all acts. Claims for illegal acts, such as inappropriate sexual behavior by a physician or teacher, are usually not covered. In some states, immunity from prosecution is provided for physicians who volunteer their time in certain settings (e.g., athletic events, clinics for indigents); teaching in these settings will also usually be shielded from prosecution.

The liability risk of teaching is usually overstated. Preceptors should have little to fear regarding their teaching activities if they are professional in their manner with patients and trainees; ask permission of patients before involving them with learners; evaluate trainees in a fair and explicit fashion; and have adequate professional liability coverage. The oversight skills, clinical currency, and intellectual stimulation provided by precepting will usually reduce a physician's overall liability and, most important, offer a rewarding and satisfying experience.

References

Kapp, M. B. 1981. Legal issues in faculty evaluation of student clinical performance. *Journal of Medical Education* 56:559–64.

Kapp, M. B. 1983. Legal implications of clinical supervision of medical students and residents. *Journal of Medical Education* 58:293–99.

Oliver, R. 1986. Legal liability of students and residents in the health care setting. *Journal of Medical Education* 61:560–68.

Roberts, R. G. 1995. Malpractice and risk management. In R. E. Rakel, ed., *Textbook of Family Practice*, 5th ed., pp. 1673–83. Philadelphia: W. B. Saunders.

Roberts, R. G., Bobula, J. A., and Wolkomir, M. 1998. Why family physicians deliver babies. *Journal of Family Practice* 46:34–40.

■ 31

Ethics of Precepting

Audrey A. Paulman, M.D., and
Jessica Pierce, Ph.D.

Key Points

- Ethical issues are a part of many clinical and teaching encounters.
- Students' ethical concerns are different from preceptors' ethical concerns.
- Each of the participants in a medical teaching encounter has a set of rights.

Formal ethics teaching, now included as part of the curriculum in most medical schools, tends to deal with issues that face practicing physicians: confidentiality of patient information, informed consent, withdrawal of life-sustaining treatment, and assisted suicide. These issues may not represent the ethical concerns of students. The student will observe the preceptor making these kinds of decisions but will probably feel like an interested third party, remote from the consequences of the choices made, and will place the intellectual and emotional responsibility for these decisions on the preceptor. On the other hand, the student will deal directly with ethical issues particular to students: practicing on patients, introducing oneself to patients, and the responsibilities of students in a health care delivery system. Since few formal ethics courses address these issues, it is important for the preceptor to help the student develop a professional sense of right and wrong.

How can the preceptor help students develop their ethical responsibilities as physicians? The preceptor needs to teach ethics explicitly, both by role modeling ethical behavior and by engaging in a dialogue with students about moral issues that arise during rotations. Mentoring has enormous power as a teaching device; it should be used consciously and with attention to what is being taught through observed behavior. The preceptor should model ethically responsible patient care. Not only do the students revere "real" physicians, they also take what they see as how things are and should be. Most medical schools offer formal ethics teaching on key topics such as confidentiality, informed consent, and respect for patient decision-making. There is also a powerful "shadow curriculum"—the things students see happening around them in the clinic, the hospital, or with their preceptor. This experience often runs counter to what they have been told in lectures. For example, students may spend the morning listening to a lecture on how all patient information must be strictly protected as confidential. They may then spend the afternoon in the hospital setting, where patient charts are lying open on the desk and physicians and students discuss patient diagnoses while standing in the hallway.

It is important for the preceptor to be sensitive to the student's level of training and help them make decisions they need to make today, not only those they need to make in the future. The preceptor can help students recognize feelings of internal conflict or confusion, which may be signs that an ethical problem may be emerging. These feelings can then be addressed as the preceptor encourages the student to look for the root of the conflict (i.e., is it training level, religious upbringing, personal choice, or patient beliefs?).

The student should then be encouraged to develop his or her own network for resolving moral conflicts. This may include such resources as formal ethics consultations, support from colleagues or other professionals, religious consultation, and family support. These sources can help the student identify both prevailing ethical standards and deeply held personal beliefs. Options can be identified and a course of action chosen.

The precepting situation also creates unique ethical responsibilities and can pose special challenges. There are four usual participants in the precepting situation: the student, the preceptor, the patient, and the medical school. Each has its own characteristics, and each has its own rights within this precepting system.

The Student's Rights

The student has a right:
■ to a productive and nourishing learning environment, where he or she is afforded a reasonable level of participation in patient care activities
■ to constructive criticism, delivered tactfully and in private
■ not to be sexually harassed or treated in an abusive manner
■ to decline participation in procedures such as abortion, with which he or she is uncomfortable for reasons of conscience
■ not to be asked to participate in activities that are illegal or contrary to professional standards
■ to decline participation in activities beyond their knowledge, skills, or capabilities

The Preceptor's Rights

The preceptor has a right:
■ to place his or her responsibility to the patient above the needs of teaching
■ to keep incompetent or unprepared students from providing care for patients (though the student

should be told why he or she is being denied participation)
- to adjust the level of participation according to each student's level of readiness and according to unique strengths and weaknesses
- to practice according to personal beliefs while making students aware of alternatives
- to have a reliable and enthusiastic student

The Patient's Rights

Patients have special rights associated with being seen in an office where medical students are precepting, including the right:
- to the confidentiality of their personal and medical information—even from the student, if requested
- to know they are being seen by a student
- to give permission to be seen by a student—and to say no
- to have their privacy respected, including freedom from sexual or inappropriately friendly relationships with caregivers
- to the best and most appropriate care

The Medical School's Rights

The medical school has a right:
- to honest feedback on student performance
- to fair grading practices by preceptors
- to know that each student will be placed in a reliable and valuable teaching setting
- to know that each student will be treated fairly and equally without regard to race, creed, gender, or disability

- to trust that preceptors will respect the students working with them and will act professionally at all times
- to know the students are in a safe environment

The precepting situation can be rewarding for everyone involved. This will be particularly true if student and preceptor alike are aware of precepting's unique ethical challenges. Preceptors who stay mindful of their role in modeling ethical behavior will perform a wonderful service for those students who spend time learning with them.

■ VII

Faculty Benefits and Resources

▪ 32

Support Services and Products Available for Community Preceptors

Daniel J. Van Durme, M.D., and
Julea Garner, M.D.

Key Points

- Community preceptors can earn continuing education credit for their efforts through the American Medical Association and the American Academy of Family Physicians.
- Faculty development programs and online resources are available for preceptors.
- A wealth of books and publications regularly discuss topics of interest to preceptors.

Community preceptors have many services and products available to assist them in teaching students and residents. Although the following discussion is not comprehensive, it includes a good sampling of materials that are of particular value to the preceptor.

Continuing Medical Education Credit

The American Academy of Family Physicians (AAFP) allows family physicians to self-report 20 continuing medical education (CME) credit hours per year of prescribed CME credits for precepting and teaching residents and medical students. This AAFP-prescribed CME credit is accepted by the American Medical Association as equivalent to AMA Category I credit for the Physicians Recognition Award. Details and online CME reporting are available for AAFP members at the AAFP Web site at <www.aafp.org>.

You can call the AAFP CME records department for more information at 1-800-274-8043.

Teaching Certificates

The AAFP Division of Education's Resident and Student Affairs/Special Projects Department produces family practice teaching certificates. Traditionally, family practice residency programs give these as an expression of their appreciation to an individual who has volunteered time and effort to teach in a family practice setting. These certificates can be displayed in the physician's office to demonstrate the importance of teaching. The family practice residency program director, the family medicine department chair, the AAFP constituent chapter, or the medical school dean may award the certificate. To qualify, an individual must have given at least 75 hours of his or her time teaching on a volunteer basis in a setting of family medicine education during the past year. Further information about teaching certificates can be obtained from the AAFP at 1-800-274-2238, ext. 5230.

Faculty Development Programs

There are specific faculty development programs for community physicians who serve as teachers. Two of the most widely used programs are the Preceptor Education Project (PEP) developed by the Society of Teachers of Family Medicine (STFM) and the Consultations in Career Development CME program developed by the AAFP Commission on Education.

The Preceptor Education Project has been consistently rated by its participants as one of the most valuable resources for specific and immediately applicable information on precepting residents and medical students. It has recently been expanded and revised as PEP2. There are three components of the program: a workshop that can be used for CME credit, a workbook that is either provided at the workshops or that can be obtained separately, and a workshop leader's manual. The workshop modules include organization and planning strategies, observation skills, teaching and feedback skills, evaluation strategies, approaches to solving problems, and a module on teaching and learning collaboratively that includes a section on informatics. A medical school, a residency program, or an AAFP constituent chapter typically sponsors the workshops. Materials and details on how to attend (or sponsor) workshops are available through the STFM at <www.stfm.org> or 1-800-274-2237, ext. 4504.

Consultations in Career Development are courses offered at the AAFP Annual Scientific Assembly (CME credit available) for family physicians who are thinking of becoming more involved in teaching and precepting. The AAFP offers several different topics each year in this area. Some courses focus on the skills and knowledge necessary to move to a faculty or management position. Other courses focus on teaching students in the office, role modeling, and developing leadership skills. Details are available through the AAFP assembly hotline at 1-800-926-6890.

Publications

There are numerous publications on precepting residents and medical students. The examples that follow are available through the STFM bookstore (1-800-274-4504 or at <www.stfm.org>). All publications in the STFM bookstore are peer reviewed to determine their usefulness and applicability for teachers of family medicine.

■ *Preceptors as Teachers: A Guide to Clinical Teaching,* 2d ed., by Neal A. Whitman and Thomas L. Schwenk. Provides "agendas" for preceptors to assess students' knowledge, attitudes, and skills.

■ *Medical Teaching and Ambulatory Care: A Practical Guide*, by Warren Rubenstein and Yves Talbot. Presents a practical approach to ambulatory care and office teaching. Covers teaching skills, office setup, how to structure a teaching day, and how to handle challenging learning situations. An excellent desktop reference.

■ *Creative Medical Training*, by Neal Whitman. Meant to inspire, not instruct, and to promote creativity in medical teaching. Topics are discussed briefly, with just enough information to encourage thinking about individual teaching.

■ The STFM journal *Family Medicine* has a regular column "For the Office-Based Teacher of Family Medicine" that offers valuable information specifically geared to the community preceptor. Past columns are available on the STFM Web site. The AAFP journal *Family Practice Management* also publishes occasional articles about office precepting.

Electronic Resources

With Internet access, you can find a vast number of resources that may improve your teaching skills and provide support. The family medicine and family practice Web sites like those of the STFM and AAFP have extensive information and more links to sites every day. Archives of information are also available via listserv at the STFM Web site. These are records of available e-mail correspondence that can be sorted for ideas and information. Listservs allow participation in e-mail discussions on topics of interest to community preceptors. One can sign up on one or more listservs to participate in these discussions. As in many aspects of our lives, the digital information age is upon us and the Internet can be used as a warehouse of information. These two Web sites can serve as librarians through their array of information.

At the local level, many medical schools and residency programs offer additional support services and rewards for local preceptors. These may include handouts and brief manuals or newsletters on how to be a better preceptor. Other benefits of precepting may include free library access, teaching aids, free computer literature searches, textbooks, stipends, or fee discounts for continuing medical education. To find out what local resources and support are available to you for precepting, contact the dean's office at your medical school, academic department, or residency program.

■ 33

Electronic Communication for Community Preceptors

Alexander W. Chessman, M.D.

Key Points

To use electronic communication in your teaching:
- Get connected to the Web.
- Show how you integrate electronic communication into your practice.
- Use the Web to improve patient care.

A critical part of a physician's job is collecting and exchanging information, and more and more information is changing hands electronically. Electronic mail connects patients to physicians, physicians to physicians, and patients to patients. Web sites are providing up-to-date information to anyone with a browser and Internet access.

Obtaining access to the Web and e-mail is an important step. Most medical schools are seeking ways both to reward community preceptors and to develop their teaching skills, and many are providing free Internet access. In addition, through advertiser funding, some organizations offer free Internet access to physicians.

Once connected to the World Wide Web, the next job is to connect to helpful information. Search engines return lists of Web sites relating to one's interest. Yahoo is an example of a general-purpose search engine <http://www.yahoo.com/>. MetaCrawler is an example of a meta-search engine that combines searches of regular search engines <http://www.metacrawler.com/>.

Another method for finding helpful Web resources is to use the links from a Web site that you like. Hardin provides a meta-directory of links for all health care <http://www.lib.uiowa.edu/hardin/md/>. Medical Matrix is another collection of links <http://www.medmatrix.org/index.asp>. Bernard Sklar maintains an annotated list of CME Web sites <http://www.medicalcomputingtoday.com/Olistcme.html>.

There are two limitations to using someone else's list. The criteria for searching and approving sites are typically not explicit. The list can also go out of date, so a good Web site will carry a notice of its most recent update. Despite these limitations, using someone else's list can be a significant time-saver.

Because Web addresses change frequently, even the most up-to-date site can list links to Web sites whose addresses have changed. If you are referred to a Web address that is no longer active, try removing the last parts of the address until you find a shorter address that works. For example, given a dead-end address such as <http://www.antihistamine.org/itch/gone/soon.html>, shorten it to <http://www.antihistamine.org/itch/gone>, or <http://www.antihistamine.org/itch>, and press enter. As a last-ditch effort, use <http://www.antihistamine.org/>, since these core addresses, or domain names, usually do not change.

Evidence-based medicine (EBM) Web sites are wonderful teaching and learning resources. The Cochrane Library is a collection of systematic reviews of therapeutic trials <http://www.jr2.ox.ac.uk/cdcig/index.html>. The *Journal of Family Practice* offers their collection of EBM reviews of articles online <http://jfp.msu.edu/jclub/jclub.htm>. Bandolier also presents reviews of clinical topics <http://www.jr2ox.ac.uk/Bandolier/band50/650-8.html>.

John Faughnan's home page <http://dragon.labmed.umn.edu/~john/index.html> provides interesting links and information on a number of health care topics.

The use of MEDLINE is a valuable skill that medical students should learn. If you are not provided access to a medical school's MEDLINE search system, then a reasonable, free option is PubMed <http://www4.ncbi.nlm.nih.gov/PubMed/>.

Electronic mail is an efficient method for communication. It is faster than a letter and avoids having to play phone tag. Patients can send a simple question that the physician can answer at his or her leisure, and no receptionist or nurse need be involved in the process.

In addition, e-mail can bring regular information updates to a physician's desktop. One example is the mailing list IAC Express. The Immunization Action Coalition and the Hepatitis B Coalition send out a newsletter about immunizations. To subscribe, send an e-mail message to <express@immunize.org> and type the word "subscribe" in the subject field.

A listserv is the equivalent of conference calls on e-mail. Listservs focus on specific content or roles. Academic-L, for example, addresses the issues facing academic physicians. Listservs are closed or open, moderated or unmoderated. Closed lists require approval of membership. Moderated lists require approval of messages before posting.

Information about specific medical conditions is available for physicians and patients on the Web. The AAFP Web site provides peer-reviewed, high-quality information <http://www.aafp.org>. The Centers for Disease Control provides extensive, up-to-date information about communicable diseases <http://www.cdc.gov/diseases/diseases.html>. An interesting site is Dr. Rose's Peripheral Brain, which consists of all the information, tips, and tricks that Dr. Rose has found useful for his own practice over the years <http://weber.u.washington.edu/~momus/PB/tableofc.htm>.

Electronic communication can improve your access to people and information. Community preceptors will find these types of interactions useful and necessary for teaching students in their practice.

▪ 34

Faculty Development

Kent J. Sheets, Ph.D.

Key Points

- ▪ Continuing faculty development will improve your teaching in the office.
- ▪ Faculty development is available through professional meetings, Web sites, and publications.

What Should I Learn?

David M. Irby, Ph.D., has been a pioneer in conducting research on teaching in the ambulatory setting. One of his studies is useful in identifying what might be the most critical skills for a community-based teacher (Irby et al., 1991). Irby's study was designed to identify the characteristics of clinical teachers in ambulatory care settings which influenced the ratings of their overall teaching effectiveness. A survey of senior medical students and medicine residents at the University of Washington in Seattle indicated that the most important characteristics of their ambulatory care teachers were (a) active involvement of the learners, (b) promotion of learner autonomy, and (c) demonstration of patient care skills. These results are consistent with those found by other investigators and suggest that developing and using these teaching behaviors is the foundation for becoming an outstanding community-based teacher.

As a community-based preceptor, you are likely to be interested in the teaching and evaluation skills required to enable you to do an excellent job teaching your medical students. Several sets of preceptor development materials have been used in workshops throughout the country in recent years, including materials prepared by the Society of Teachers of Family Medicine (STFM) Preceptor Education Project (PEP) (1st ed., 1992; 2d ed., PEP2, 1999) and the Primary Care Futures Project (PCFP) (Massachusetts Statewide AHEC Program, 1996). A review of the table of contents for these materials can give you an idea of what skills you should have as a preceptor.

In the PEP materials, organization and planning, observation, teaching, feedback, evaluation, and handling problems are identified as core precepting skills. In the second edition of the PEP, teaching and learning collaboratively and assessment have been added. PEP materials can be obtained from STFM, P.O. Box 7370, Shawnee Mission, Kans. 66207-0370 (1-800-274-2237).

The PCFP faculty development materials have been used extensively in multispecialty and multidisciplinary workshops for faculty in community health centers and other community settings. The PCFP materials emphasize the characteristics of the effective teacher, the components of an educational planning process, and different teaching styles and methods. They also describe how to conduct educational evaluations, in particular how to provide feedback to the learner.

As part of the educational planning process, the mnemonic GNOME is used. GNOME reminds the preceptor to consider *g*oals, *n*eeds (of the learner), *o*bjectives, *m*ethods (of instruction), and *e*valuation during each encounter with a student. The teaching styles and methods that are proposed are categorized as assertive, suggestive, collaborative, and facilitative.

PCFP materials can be obtained from the University of Massachusetts Medical Center, Community Faculty Development Center, Suite A3-148 Benedict Building, 55 Lake Avenue N, Worcester, Mass. 01655 (508-856-1643).

Where and How Should I Learn?

There are many sources of preceptor development activities. The challenge is to find the sources that are the most accessible to you and activities that are compatible with your situation and preferred learning style. These sources include:

- the school or department that assigns students to you
- the students
- self-study
- national and state specialty academy-sponsored activities and materials
- health system-sponsored activities and materials

The School or Department That Assigns Students to You

Your initial source of faculty development to support your teaching of medical students should be the medical school or department that assigns students to work in your practice. Most teaching programs have preceptor manuals or handbooks that outline the basic preceptor requirements. These manuals often contain faculty development tips or opportunities as well as details on how the clerkship or preceptorship functions.

The school or department should provide regular faculty development via site visits to your practice or workshops on campus. Articles or other materials, such as the *Family Medicine* column "For the Office-Based Teacher of Family Medicine," may be helpful.

The Students

The medical students assigned to your practice are also a potential source of faculty development. Community-based teachers often take advantage of the students' recent immersion in the academic medical center to learn the latest approach to the treatment of specific diseases. Preceptors can also benefit from the students' experience with computer and other information technology and improve their own teaching and self-directed learning skills. Students can also describe teaching techniques they have found useful in other clerkships that the preceptor might be encouraged to try as well.

Self-Study

If you obtain most of your continuing medical education by means of self-study methods (audiotapes, journal articles, Internet-based materials, etc.), then you might be likely to use self-study to develop your precepting skills. Numerous books, journals, and other resources are described in Chapter 32 on support services and products for community preceptors. If you have Internet access, you can develop your skills as a teacher by exploring the various preceptor development materials that are available in print, in various audiovisual media, and in cyberspace.

National and State Academy-Sponsored Activities and Materials

There are several venues for developing teaching skills through nationally sponsored activities and materials. Readily available materials to develop preceptorship include the PEP and PCFP materials mentioned earlier. In addition to specialty-specific organizations such as the American Academy of Family Physicians (AAFP), American Academy of Pediatrics (AAP), or American College of Physicians (ACP), there are more broadly based organizations such as the National Health Service Corps (NHSC) and the National Rural Health Association (NRHA) which have incorporated sessions on teaching skills into their national meetings or their publications. An example of a publication prepared by a specialty organization is *Community-Based Teaching*, published by the ACP (Deutsch and Noble, 1997).

The beauty of including sessions on teaching skills in these meetings is that it enables physicians to combine development of their clinical and teaching skills. For example, each year many family physicians attend workshops at the AAFP Scientific Assembly to develop and enhance their teaching skills. One to two workshops on teaching students in the office are routinely offered at this national meeting.

Several organizations are geared more toward academic physicians but offer programs or materials for use by the community-based teacher. These include the STFM, the Ambulatory Pediatric Association (APA), and the Society of General Internal Medicine (SGIM). A publication from pediatrics entitled *Pediatric Education in Community Settings: A Manual* was published as a joint effort involving the AAP and APA (DeWitt and Roberts, 1996). The STFM provides scholarships for community preceptors to attend some of their national and regional meetings as a means to improve interactions between academic family physicians and their community colleagues.

For some preceptors, there are opportunities at the local and regional level. Some state academies sponsor preceptor development programs as part of state or regional meetings.

Activities and Materials Sponsored by Health Systems

In areas of the country where health systems have made a commitment to supporting education, the health systems have sometimes supported teaching development programs for the system's physicians. As more medical schools enter into collaborative relationships with health systems, this might become a more frequent source of preceptor development activities.

As you develop your strategy for improving your teaching skills, you will note that continuing medical education (CME) credit is often provided for some of the faculty development activities. This might be a criterion in choosing your development activities. Another point to consider as you develop your teaching skills is their value to role modeling and mentoring. If you are a relatively inexperienced preceptor, you should consider contacting former preceptors or role models of your own to ask them for help as you begin your own precepting. Or conversely, if you are an experienced preceptor, be responsive to those less experienced preceptors who ask you questions about issues they confront in their early efforts.

A wide range of options are available to you in your efforts to develop your teaching skills. Your specialty, your geographic location, and the nature of your affiliation with a medical school or health system will dictate some of your options for continued development of your teaching skills. Contact your medical school or department to further explore the options available to you.

References

Deutsch, S. L., and Noble, J. (eds.). 1997. *Community-Based Teaching*. Philadelphia: American College of Physicians.

DeWitt, T. G., and Roberts, B. (eds.). 1996. *Pediatric Education in Community Settings: A Manual*. Arlington, Va.: National Center for Education in Maternal and Child Health.

Irby, D. M., Ramsey, P. G., Gillmore, G. M., and Schaad, D. 1991. Characteristics of effective clinical teachers of ambulatory care medicine. *Academic Medicine* 66:54–55.

Massachusetts Statewide AHEC Program. 1996. *The Primary Care Futures Project Faculty Development Curriculum: A Multi-disciplinary Curriculum and Resource Guide for Teaching in Community Health Centers*. Massachusetts Statewide AHEC Program, University of Massachusetts Medical Center, Worcester, Mass.

Society of Teachers of Family Medicine. 1992. *Preceptor Education Project (PEP) Workshop Materials*. Society of Teachers of Family Medicine, Kansas City, Mo.

Society of Teachers of Family Medicine. 1999. *Preceptor Education Project Workshop Materials*. 2d ed. (PEP2) Workshop Materials. Society of Teachers of Family Medicine, Kansas City, Mo.

▪ Appendix A

Health Care Financing Administration Rules for Student Documentation in Medicare Patients' Charts

Medical Student Documentation. Medical student documentation for evaluation and management services, i.e., the review of systems (ROS) and past family and social history (PFSH), may be referred to and utilized by the teaching physician (TP), but not the student's documentation relative to physical exam. The TP must perform the physical exam and document the key elements in order to bill a fee (memorandum from R. Dickler, Division of Health Care Affairs, Association of American Medical Colleges, Feb. 3, 1997).

Sample Preceptor-University Contract

An Agreement between the Department of (name of department, ex. family practice)
School of Medicine
XXXXXXXXXXXX University
and XXXXX(1) XXXXX(2), XXXXX(3) (hereinafter "Preceptor").

WHEREAS, the University has a curriculum leading to a doctoral degree in medicine; and

WHEREAS, clinical education and experience are required and integral components of that curriculum; and

WHEREAS, the University desires the assistance of the Preceptor in developing and implementing the first- and second-year clinical education program in generalist medicine (family practice, general internal medicine, and general pediatrics); and

WHEREAS, the University further desires that its medical students receive instruction in and learn the highest standards of generalist medicine through study and teaching in medical practices in urban, rural, and suburban settings; and

WHEREAS, the Preceptor wishes to assist the University in developing and implementing clinical education and experience in generalist medicine for the University's first- and second-year medical students.

NOW, THEREFORE, the parties agree as follows:

I. *Responsibilities of the Preceptor*

A. The Preceptor must meet the criteria for selection as described in the addendum to this Agreement.

B. The Preceptor, as an independent contractor, will provide clinical instruction and supervision to first- and/or second-year medical student(s) for the course, "Foundations of Clinical Medicine," in the Preceptor's clinical setting.

C. For each student assigned to the Preceptor, the Preceptor will teach 15, three-hour sessions between the hours of 1:00 and 5:00 P.M., twice per month, per student, beginning in August/September and concluding in April/May. Any teaching services provided in addition to the foregoing sessions will be considered volunteer services for which no compensation will be paid by the University.

D. The Preceptor will follow a prescribed curriculum as stated in written curricular guidelines provided by the University.

E. The Preceptor will have ultimate responsibility for providing care to the recipients of his or her or its services (hereinafter referred to as "patients").

F. The Preceptor will provide qualified staff, patients, physical facilities, clinical equipment, and materials in accordance with preceptorship objectives as agreed upon by the Preceptor and the University.

G. The Preceptor will provide each assigned student with appropriate supervision during the preceptorship experience.

H. The Preceptor will provide each assigned student with an orientation to the Preceptor site, including a copy of pertinent rules and regulations pertaining to the Preceptor site.

I. The Preceptor will evaluate the performance of each assigned student in writing, using forms provided or approved by the University. Evaluation materials will be forwarded or delivered to the University within three weeks of the conclusion of the student's preceptorship assignment at the Preceptor site.

J. The Preceptor will advise the University at the earliest possible time of any changes in operation, policies, or personnel that may affect the clinical teaching services provided pursuant to this Agreement.

K. The Preceptor will advise the University at the earliest possible time of any serious deficiency noted in an assigned student's performance. If practicable, and in consultation with the student, the Preceptor and the University will devise a plan by which the student may be assisted toward achieving the stated objectives of the preceptorship experience.

L. The Preceptor reserves the right to request, upon written notice to the University, that the University withdraw from the preceptorship any student whose performance is detrimental to patient well-being or to the achievement of the stated objectives of the preceptorship experience.

II. *Responsibilities of the University*

A. The University will maintain communication with the Preceptor on matters pertinent to clinical education. Such communication may include, but is not limited to, visits to the Preceptor site, requests that the Preceptor attend workshops or meetings related to clinical education, and the provision of educational materials relevant to the clinical education program.

B. The University will advise students assigned to the Preceptor of their responsibility for complying with the existing rules and regulations of the Preceptor.

C. The University will maintain liability insurance for each student assigned to the Preceptor and will provide the Preceptor with information regarding such liability insurance upon request.

D. The University will notify the Preceptor of its planned

schedule for each student assignment, including the dates of preceptorship experience, the name(s) of each student, and the level of academic and preclinical preparation of each student.

E. The University will provide the Preceptor with educational objectives and evaluation forms for the preceptorship experience.

F. The University reserves the right to withdraw a student from a preceptorship assignment upon written notice to the Preceptor, if the University determines that conditions at the Preceptor site are not beneficial to student learning.

III. *Responsibilities of the Student*

A. The University will inform students that they are responsible for demonstrating professional behavior appropriate to the environment at the Preceptor site, including protecting the confidentiality of patient information and maintaining high standards of patient care.

B. A student has the right to request withdrawal from a preceptorship assignment for cause, upon written notice to the University. Said notice shall state the reason(s) for the request. The University, in its sole discretion, shall determine whether the request will be granted.

IV. *Term*   This Agreement shall commence on (date) and end on (date). At the end of said initial term, this Agreement shall be automatically renewed for a one-year term unless either party provides notice of nonrenewal at least thirty (30) days before the end of the initial term. Notwithstanding any provision to the contrary, either party may terminate this Agreement at any time upon at least thirty (30) days' written notice to the other, provided that any student(s) currently assigned to the Preceptor at the time of notice of termination shall be given the opportunity to complete his or her or their preceptorship experience at the Preceptor site, such completion not to exceed three months.

V. *Notice*   Any written communication or notice pursuant to this Agreement shall be made to the following representatives of the respective parties at the following addresses:
For the University:
Name
Department
Address
City, State, ZIP
Phone
For the Preceptor:
Preceptor Name
Preceptor Address

VI. *Severability*   If any provision of this Agreement is held to be invalid or unenforceable for any reason, this Agreement shall remain in full force and effect in accordance with its terms, with the exception of such unenforceable or invalid provision.

VII. *Agreement Headings*   The headings contained herein are used solely for convenience and shall not be deemed to limit or define the provisions of this Agreement.

VIII. *No Waiver*   Any failure of a party to enforce that party's rights under any provision of this Agreement shall not be construed or act as a waiver of said party's subsequent right to enforce any of the provisions contained herein.

IX. *Entire Understanding*   This Agreement contains the entire understanding of the parties as to the matters contained herein, and it shall not be altered, amended, or modified except in writing executed by the duly authorized officials of both the University and the Preceptor.

X. *Governing Law*   This agreement shall be governed and construed in accordance with existing state and federal statutes.

In witness whereof the parties have caused this Agreement to be duly executed, effective as herein set forth.

By _____   _____
     Preceptor   Date

By _____   _____
     XXXXXX, M.D.   Date
     Vice President for
     Health Sciences

By _____   _____
     XXXXXX, M.D.   Date
     Chair, Department
     of Family Practice

Contract Addendum—Criteria for Selection

Criteria for preceptors for the course, "(title of course)," are as follows:

1. positive reputation and recommendations as a competent teacher, clinician, and role model

2. previous teaching or precepting experience as evaluated by students or residents

3. an M.D. or D.O. degree and primary care practice in family practice, general internal medicine, or general pediatrics; medical board certification or eligibility for board certification is preferred

4. a license to practice medicine in (name of state) and current good standing with the board of medicine

5. availability and willingness to precept students on Wednesday or Thursday afternoons for first-year students and Tuesday or Wednesday afternoons for second-year students

6. location of practice within a sixty (60)-minute commute from (name of city and state) unless special circumstances exist for the use of a more distant practice

Index

Library of Congress Cataloging-in-Publication Data

Precepting medical students in the office / edited by Paul M.
Paulman, Jeffrey L. Susman, Cheryl A. Abboud.
     p. ; cm.
  Includes bibliographical references and index.
  ISBN 0-8018-6366-X (pbk : alk. paper)
  1. Medicine—Study and teaching (Preceptorship). 2. Primary
care (Medicine)—Study and teaching. 3. Ambulatory medical
care—Study and teaching. I. Paulman, Paul M., 1953–
II. Susman, Jeffrey. III. Abboud, Cheryl A., 1961–
[DNLM: 1. Preceptorship—methods. 2. Students, Medical.
W 20 P923 2000]
R837.P74 P74 2000
610'.71'1—dc21   99-052722